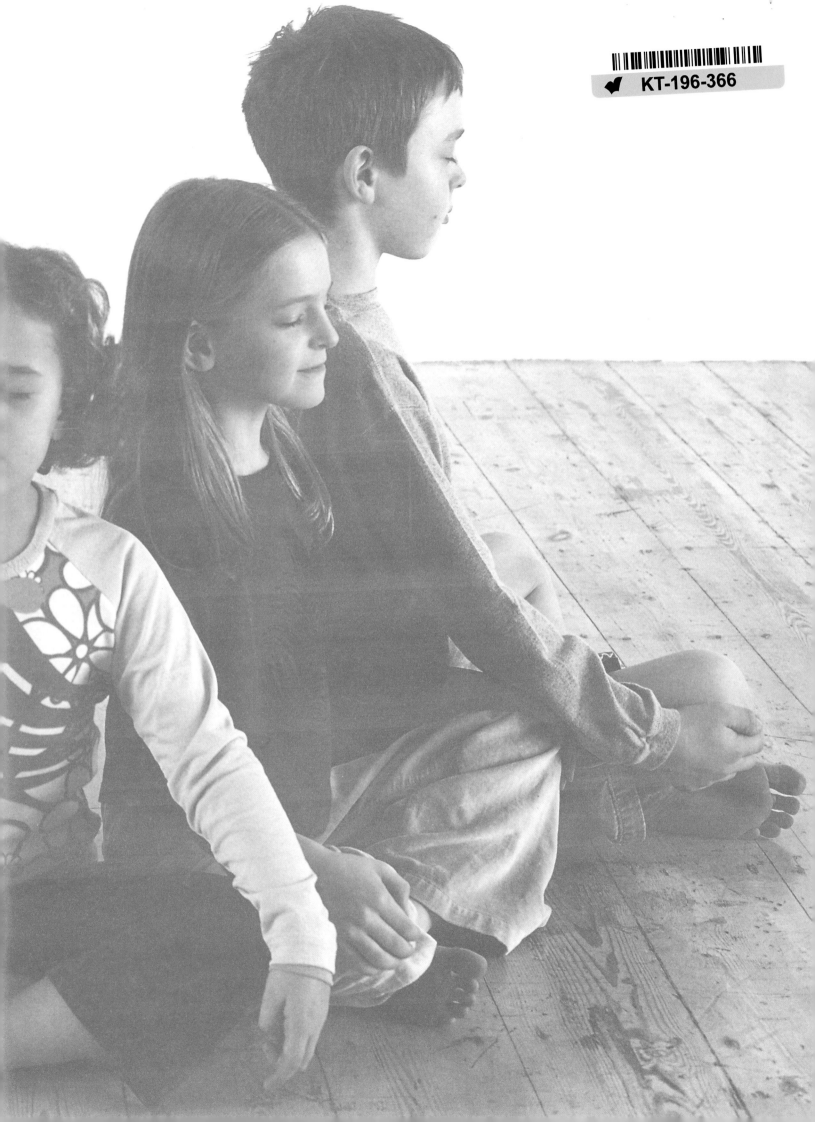

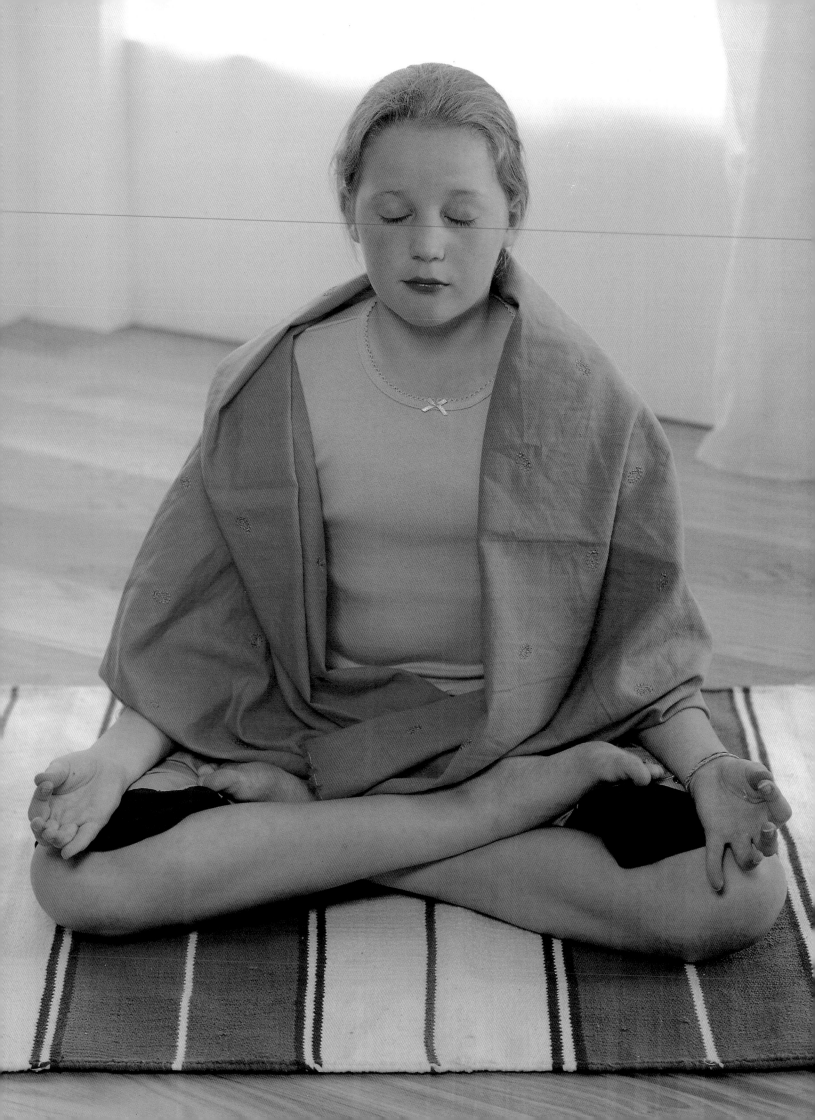

Yoga
for children

Stretching and
strengthening exercises
for 3-11 year olds

Bel Gibbs

LORENZ BOOKS

Dedication

To lovely Linda, who got me started on my yoga journey and who shares in my adventures...

This edition is published by Lorenz Books

Lorenz Books is an imprint of Anness Publishing Ltd,
Hermes House, 88–89 Blackfriars Road, London SE1 8HA
tel. 020 7401 2077; fax 020 7633 9499
www.lorenzbooks.com; info@anness.com

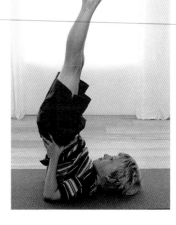

This edition distributed in the UK by The Manning Partnership Ltd, 6 The Old Dairy, Melcombe Road, Bath BA2 3LR;
tel. 01225 478 444; fax 01225 478 440; sales@manning-partnership.co.uk

This edition distributed in the USA and Canada by National Book Network, 4720 Boston Way, Lanham, MD 20706;
tel. 301 459 3366; fax 301 459 1705; www.nbnbooks.com

This edition distributed in Australia by Pan Macmillan Australia, Level 18, St Martins Tower, 31 Market St, Sydney,
NSW 2000; tel. 1300 135 113; fax 1300 135 103; customer.service@macmillan.com.au

This edition distributed in New Zealand by David Bateman Ltd, 30 Tarndale Grove, Off Bush Road, Albany,
Auckland; tel. (09) 415 7664; fax (09) 415 8892

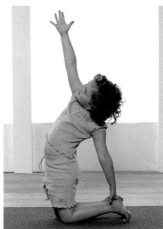

A CIP catalogue record for this book is available from the British Library.

Publisher: **Joanna Lorenz**
Managing Editor: **Judith Simons**
Project Editor: **Sarah Ainley**
Photographer: **John Freeman**
Additional Photography: **Clare Park**
Photography stylist: **Sue Duckworth**
Designer: **Lisa Tai**
Illustrator: **Lucy Grossmith**
Production Controller: **Claire Rae**

10 9 8 7 6 5 4 3 2 1

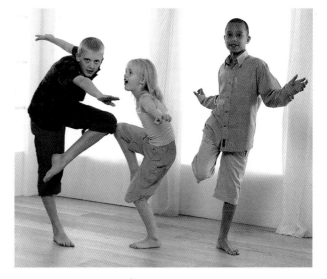

Contents

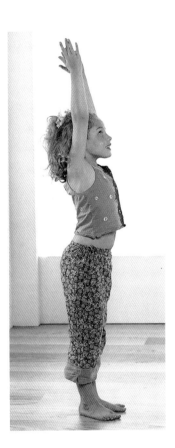

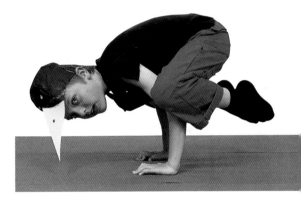

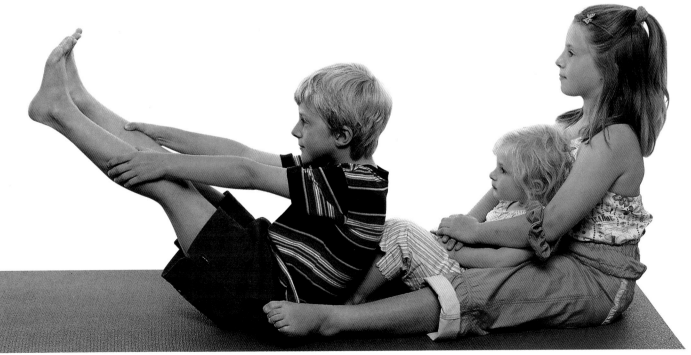

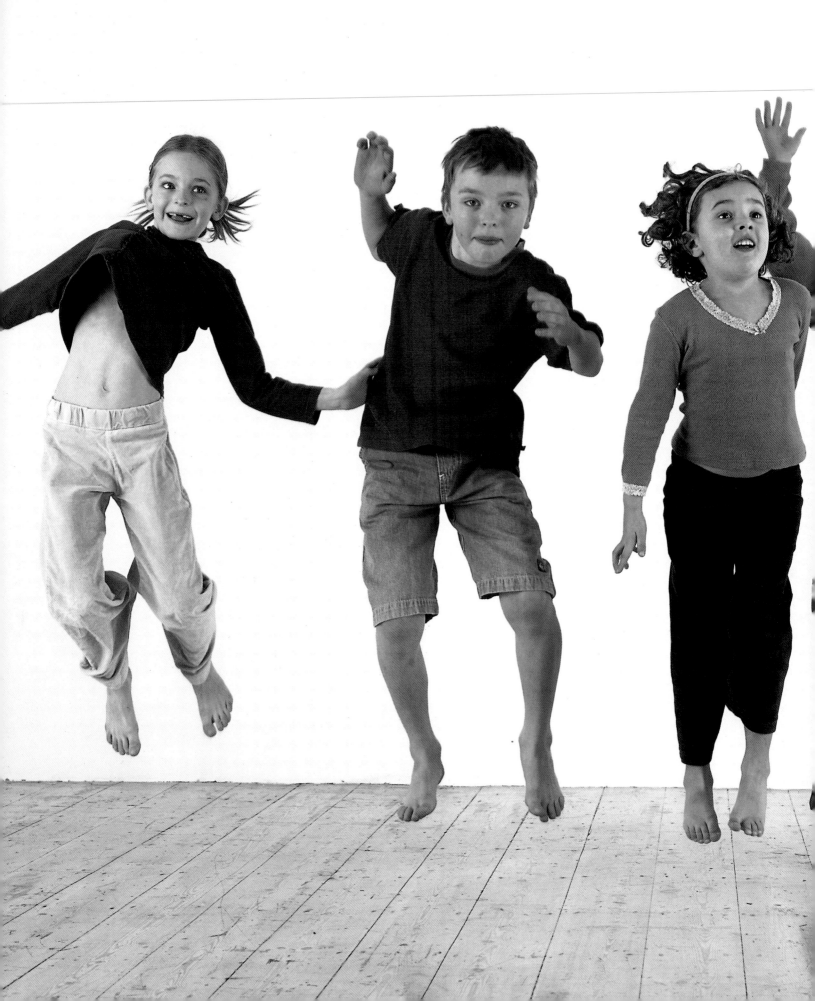

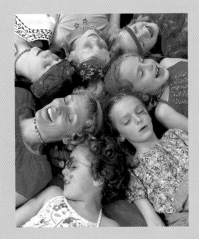

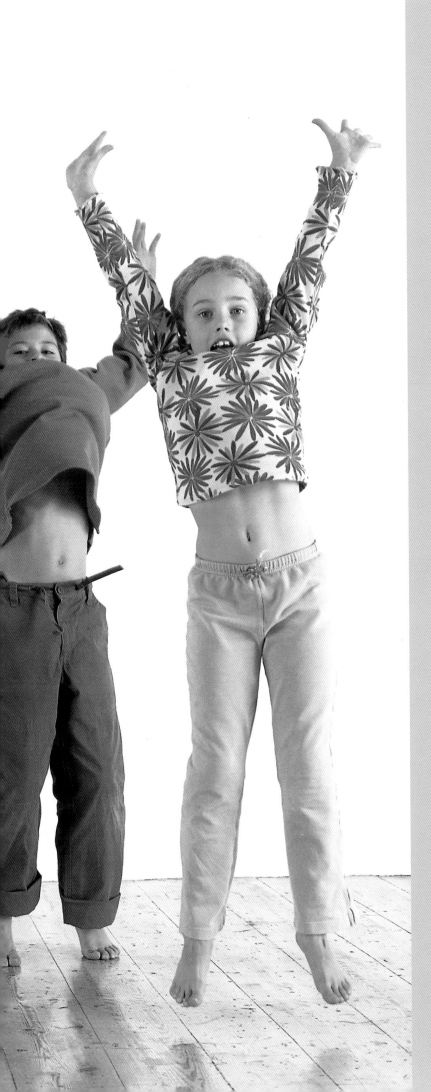

introduction

The following pages will inspire you to put yoga firmly on your family agenda. A brief history "lesson" explains how yoga began and why the yoga philosophy for health and well-being is still relevant to our busy lives today. We all have a special place inside us that that holds the key to our inner potential, like a treasure chest of precious jewels, and here we show children how to unlock their own inner powers. Simply follow the fun and simple warm-up exercises to get you started, and your yoga journey will have truly begun.

Welcome to your very own yoga book

introduction

Adults have been practising yoga for many years, and while many people complain that children today are growing up too fast, yoga is something they can never start too young. Introducing the concept and practice of yoga and a yogic lifestyle to your children means that you are giving them the very best start in life.

yoga for children

Childhood is a vibrant time when natural energy and creativity are high, also when eyes and minds are open and learning is fun. This makes it the perfect time for children to explore and enjoy their bodies, while putting them in touch with how their minds' work and introducing them to the idea of an inner self, or soul.

We all have the potential to develop our inner self, and yoga can show us how. Yoga is expressive, and this is

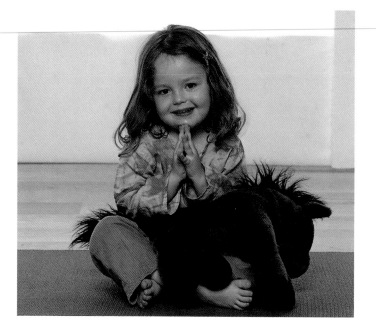

◁ Yoga encourages us to find quiet time and to enjoy being rather than doing.

what makes it so appealing to children. There are countless benefits of yoga for children, but the principal focus is to nurture a strong, healthy body, a calm, contented mind and, with commitment, a sense of inner peace.

what's in it for parents?

This yoga book is primarily aimed at children between the ages of 3 and 11 years, but in a sense it is for children of all ages. As you demonstrate the yoga postures to your children, you will be rekindling your own sense of fun, putting you in touch with your inner child. You will also be increasing your motivation as a parent by taking an active role in the well-being of your child, physically, emotionally and spiritually. By practising yoga as a family, you will be spending valuable time together, learning new skills and having fun, and all without having to go near a television or the car!

what's in this book?

This book is written with a sense of fun and adventure. It is bursting with animals and objects from the natural

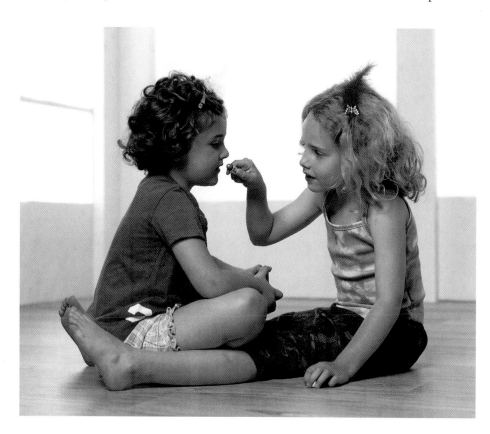

◁ Enjoying spending time with family and friends is an important part of growing up and will help us to build lasting relationships later on in life.

world, all of which will appeal instinctively to a child's imagination. So this is where we start. Encourage your child to "become" an animal from the colourful, easy to follow Animal Parade chapter. As they become adept at the animal postures, try some of the other fun poses and encourage your children to make up their own, or link them together in the themed story sequences in the Putting It All Together chapter. Try some of the yoga games, and even act out a yoga play. There are also ideas on how to organize a child's birthday party with a yoga theme.

In addition, learn how yoga breathing exercises can alter your children's moods and how peaceful postures, chanting and meditating can soothe away tension and nurture quiet time and contemplation.

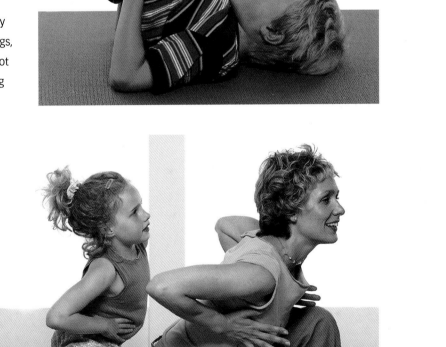

◁ Yoga postures can help you to view things from a different perspective.

◁ The thought of imitating the behaviour and movements of their favourite animals is most children's idea of a lot of fun!

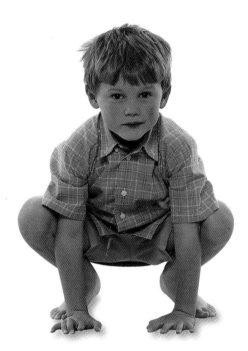

▽ Crow walking helps to physically strengthen our legs, and teaches us not to take everything too seriously.

Where does yoga come from?

Yoga evolved several thousand years ago, in India, as a system of self-enlightenment. Today, in spite of all the benefits of 21st-century living, more and more people are turning to yoga for inspiration, and this confirms its timeless appeal.

the meaning of yoga

Originally, yoga evolved as a way of feeling closer to a higher, divine presence, and the focus of yoga practice was spiritual rather than physical. Today, yoga can be enjoyed as a physical discipline, known as Hatha yoga, as well as a spiritual one. Indeed, many people find that practising yoga can help to deepen their faith.

The gurus who first developed the idea of yoga believed that to attain spiritual enlightenment required a systematic approach. They devised a code of practice for all-round health, and believed that by training the physical body – the first step in Hatha yoga – they could tame the mind, improve concentration, and find their inner self or soul.

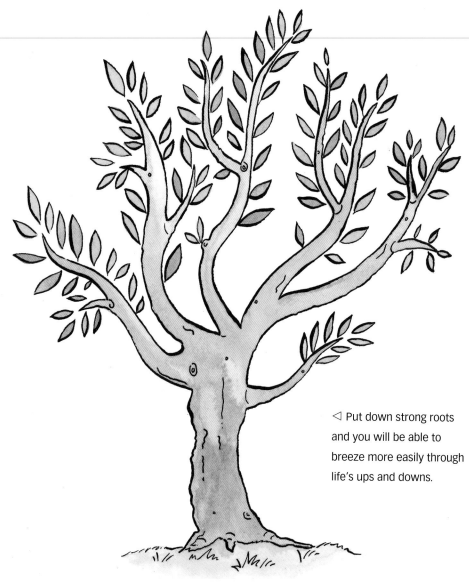

◁ Put down strong roots and you will be able to breeze more easily through life's ups and downs.

nature knows best

The gurus sought their initial inspiration from the natural world around them. They watched and studied the patterns of nature and the behaviour of animals with a scientific passion. They marvelled at the power and focus of predatory creatures and birds as they hunted, at their ability to conserve energy and to sleep soundly when the opportunity arose.

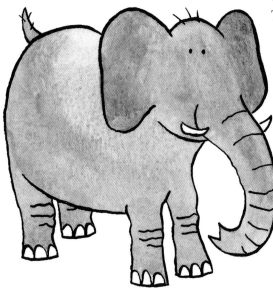

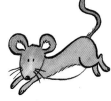

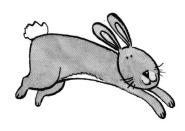

◁ ▷ Some animals inspire us with their quick agility, while others show it pays to take things slow.

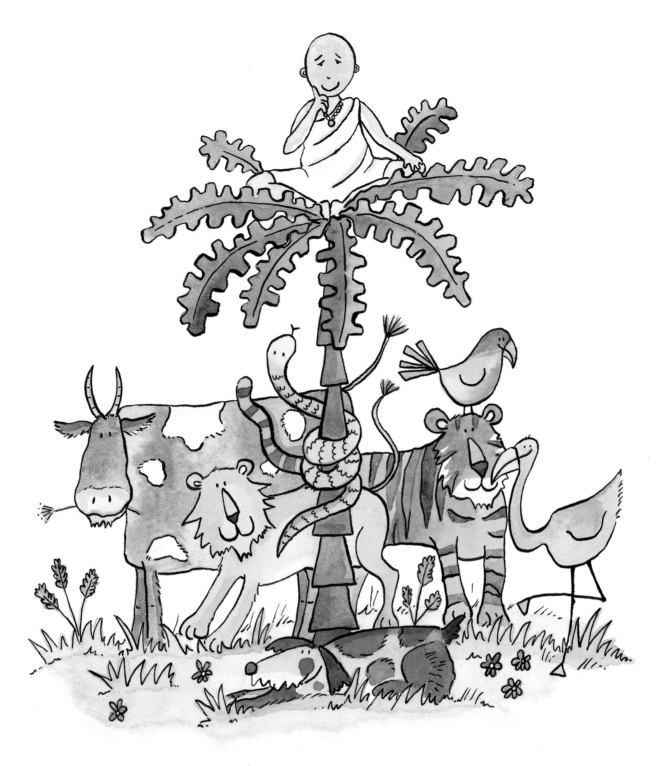

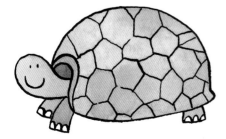

Admiring this balanced, instinctive way of living, the yogis – the gurus who developed and practised the yoga philosophy – began to imitate the way the animals moved and behaved, and soon they found themselves empowered with special qualities. And so the classical asanas or animal postures were born.

what the yogis learned

The gurus observed the breathing patterns of animals, and noted that animals with slow heart rates, like the elephant and the tortoise, lived much longer than agile and nervous animals with quick heart rates, such as mice and rabbits.

They saw the sun as the centre of their energy universe after watching how plants and flowers grow upwards

△ Just like the yogis of ancient times, you can learn from the natural world around you. Simply open your eyes and strive to see the good in everything.

to bask in its warmth and energy. They admired the huge trees because they were at the same time strong and flexible, rooted firmly in the ground but with branches moving freely in the wind. Seeing these attributes as metaphors for a human code of living, they saw that man could be happier and healthier if he, too, could be both grounded and flexible.

Yoga and your body

According to yoga philosophy, a human being is made up of different layers, a bit like an onion. There are three of these layers, and they are known as koshas.

you are an onion!

The first layer is our physical body, called the *annamaya kosha*. This is the layer we are most familiar with because it is visible and we use it for all our everyday activities. The second layer is our mind or mental layer, or *manamaya kosha*. This is where our thoughts, feelings and emotions take place. The third is our spiritual layer, or *anandamaya kosha*, and this is the home of our inner self or soul.

The mental and spiritual layers are more difficult to relate to because they are invisible, but the aim of yoga is to use our physical body as a way of reaching first the mental and then the spiritual layer. It is here that yogis believe true happiness resides, and if we can reach our inner self we can enjoy a whole new side of our personality. Regular yoga practice can help to connect us with the inner self and develop our spiritual nature. The sooner we start on this wonderful inward journey the better.

getting physical

The human body is made up of a brain, a heart, two lungs, trillions of tiny cells, 206 bones, 600 muscles and lots of blood. More than half our body weight is made up of water. The brain is the body's central computer, delivering instructions and messages to the limbs and internal organs, while the heart is a powerful pump pushing blood around the body. The blood is

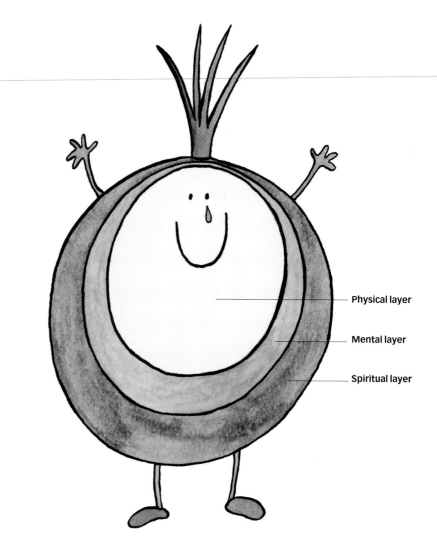

our body's "river of life", transporting its precious cargo of oxygen and nutrients to where they are needed, and relaying waste and carbon dioxide back to our lungs to be breathed away. Our lungs are like two big sponges that soak up oxygen from the air we breathe to keep us alive. As for all that water inside us, this is absolutely vital as every bodily function from swallowing and blinking to breathing and moving – including reading this book – needs water.

Our bones are like scaffolding bound together by bandage-like muscles that literally stop us from falling apart. If our muscles are too tight, we feel stiff and our movements are limited. If left for long periods of

Physical layer

Mental layer

Spiritual layer

△ Think of all the parts that go into the layering of an onion. The more parts you unravel, the more there seems to be. This is the wonder of you too!

time, tight muscles can affect our physical posture and how we carry ourselves, locking our bodies into uncomfortable positions and leading to rounded shoulders, stiff necks and knock knees. The good news is that muscles can be retrained through gentle, regular stretching, which helps them to regain their elasticity. This allows us to straighten our shoulders and open up our chests, stand tall with our heads up, touch our toes with ease, avoid injuries and generally feel in good physical shape.

why it is wise to exercise

The benefits of physical exercise are enormous. Exercise strengthens the heart, and this promotes good circulation, which increases the flow of oxygen- and nutrient-rich blood to all parts of the body. Boosting the circulation speeds up the elimination of waste products, improves digestion, and helps to relax tense muscles, releasing mental stress and negative emotions. Exercise also strengthens bones, tones muscles and ligaments, keeping us trim and fit. It increases energy levels and produces endorphins, the body's natural feel-good hormones, which enhance mood and well-being.

All types of exercise are good in moderation, but a variety of activities will work a wider range of muscles. Introducing yoga as a complement to regular exercise is manageable because it can be done at home and it doesn't cost anything. Because yoga can involve all members of the family, it offers valuable bonding time while teaching important new life skills.

hatha yoga

Physical or Hatha yoga forms the essence of this book and relates to the practice of special postures called asanas. These asanas have evolved to work all parts of the body. They fall into families of postures, including forward bends, backward bends, standing poses, seated poses, twists, side-bending postures, balances and inverted postures. As you work through the book you will see that the groups of postures have different physical and emotional effects. Some are calming and grounding, while others are energizing and uplifting.

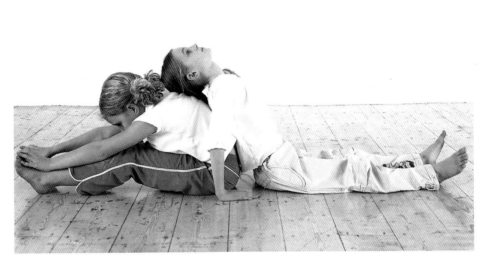

△ We can use our bodies in so many ways. This assisted Sandwich pose quietens the mind as you fold your upper body forwards, and it gives your partner a nice back stretch at the same time.

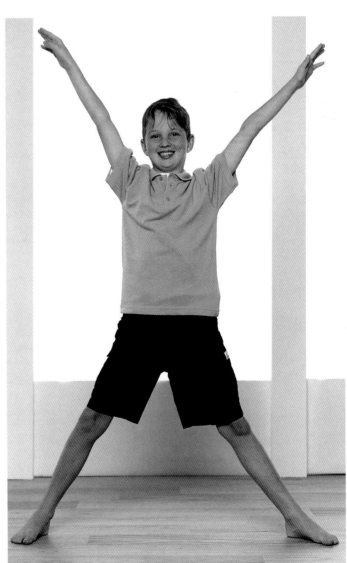

▷ The body is your temple and physical activity makes your body an exhilarating place to live in.

What's on your mind?

In yoga philosophy, the mind is the body's second layer. It is the force that both drives the physical body and feeds our inner world or soul, where the yogis believe our true nature is to be found. The mind plays an essential role in determining whether our journey through life will be smooth or bumpy, or whether our glass will be half full or half empty.

The guru Patanjali defined yoga as "the mastery of the stilling of the mind". He believed in training the mind to focus completely on one thing at a time and therefore become as useful as possible.

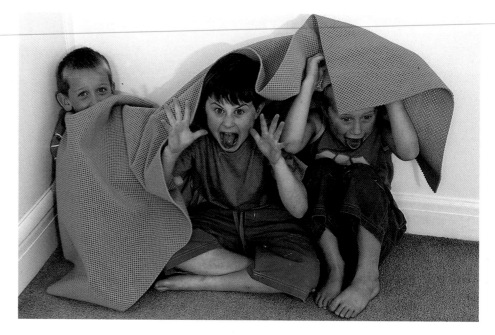

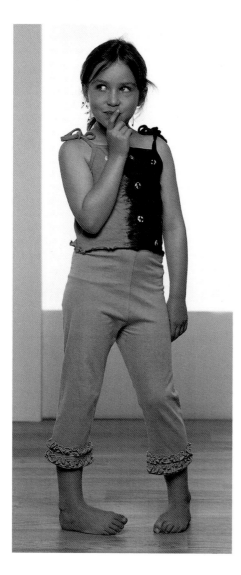

five ways of thinking

The gurus who developed yoga philosophy believed that our thought processes functioned at five different levels, from muddled and irrational to clear and focused. The latter, superior level of thinking is attainable by all of us, but we first have to conquer the lower thought processes that govern our irrational or base behaviour.

Our least refined level of thinking is likened to a drunken monkey swinging from branch to branch, where thoughts are random and jumpy with no common thread. Moving up, the second level resembles a lethargic water buffalo standing in the mud, inactive and uninspired. The third level – which is the most common mental state – is a mobile mind that flits endlessly between doubt and conviction, knowing and not knowing. The fourth level reveals a relatively clear mind that has

△ Give it a rest! A mind that is always busy can become physically exhausting.

direction but lacks attention. The fifth and highest level is where the mind is linked exclusively with the object of its attention. Here, mind and object unite and merge to become one.

minding the mind

Learning to refine our thinking processes is one of the rewards of regular yoga practice. The yoga techniques outlined in this book concentrate on yoga postures, breath awareness and learning to enjoy stillness and silence. Getting to grips with these essential techniques will help you to improve your ability to concentrate. This is the first stage in learning to control the endless fluctuations of the mind.

why concentrate?

The art of concentration is being lost. It is being undermined by the desire to be permanently busy and a notion

◁ Thinking before you speak or act helps you to behave appropriately.

that we must always be achieving, producing and progressing. So involved are we in multi-tasking that we risk becoming a jack of all trades but master of none. The absence of concentration makes it difficult for us to sit still, or think before we speak, or plan before we act. Those unruly monkeys take over our mind and our physical body responds with restless behaviour and hyperactivity.

present and correct

Concentration helps us to enjoy the "bloom" of the present moment and to think about tomorrow only when tomorrow comes; this is how it feels to be absorbed in a good book or enjoy an interesting conversation with a friend. Concentration makes for attentiveness in school and the ability to understand and retain information. It lets us fully engage with the people around us, and helps to cement relationships. It allows us to put 100 per cent of ourselves into

everything we do, and means we will always do our best. In the same way that the sun's rays can be intensified through a magnifying glass, our fragmented thoughts can be harnessed together to make a powerful tool.

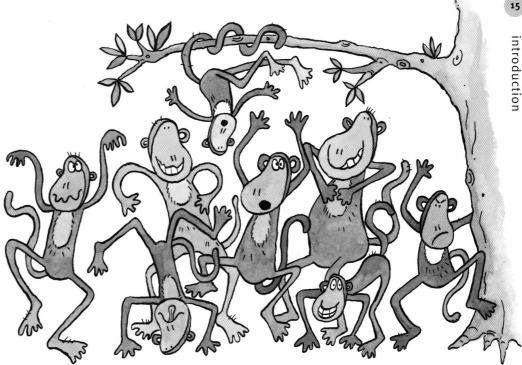

△ Left to its own devices the mind can become as unruly as these monkeys.

meditation

Once we have learned how to concentrate and focus our mind and energies on one thing at a time, we can begin to talk about meditation. Meditation is simply concentration in a more *concentrated* form. Think of concentration as a flow of water that stops and starts. Meditation is simply a flow of water that continues unbroken in an endless stream.

One way or another, we are all looking for the peace of mind that this deeper level of concentration brings. When our attention is fully engaged, our mind becomes silent, worries are temporarily forgotten and an inner contentment replaces all else.

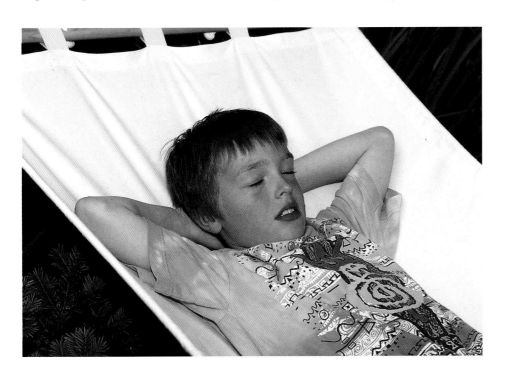

◁ The inner contentment that a quiet mind brings is available to all of us.

Your invisible friend the breath

Breathing is our most important daily activity and, alongside eating, it is one of the two ways in which we provide our body with the energy it needs to live. That said, we can live for a few days without eating but only a few moments without breathing. Learning to be aware of, and improve, our habitual breathing patterns can dynamically enhance our physical, mental and emotional well-being.

Regular breathing encourages the exchange of old air for new. Breathing in and out through the nose involves complete in and out breaths, which encourage the diaphragm to contract and relax, massaging the heart and all of the abdominal organs respectively.

Shallow breathing, on the other hand, robs the lungs of oxygen and the diaphragm of its potential range of movement. With the lungs unable to function properly, stale air can become trapped and the body is deprived of oxygen. This is when our resistance to illness drops.

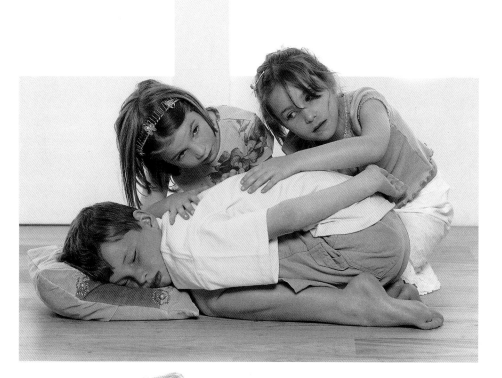

△ Finding the breath. All children will enjoy the challenge of trying to find something they cannot see.

◁ Look, no hands! Blowing a feather demonstrates the power of the breath – something we all take for granted.

posture
Diaphragmatic breathing, or tummy breathing, opens up the chest and allows the lungs to expand. We all have to stand tall or sit upright to breathe in this way. This means that our chest opens, our shoulders drop and overall posture is modified for the better. All in all, good breathing habits produce a stronger respiratory system, improved posture and a happier frame of mind.

prana
In yoga philosophy, the other function of breathing is to increase our vital life energy, known as *prana*. The yogis believed that this in turn would lead to control of the mind.

Prana is controlled by special breathing exercises or *pranayama* (*ayama* meaning to lengthen or add a new dimension to). These exercises are designed to enhance our life energy and help us connect to our quiet inner self.

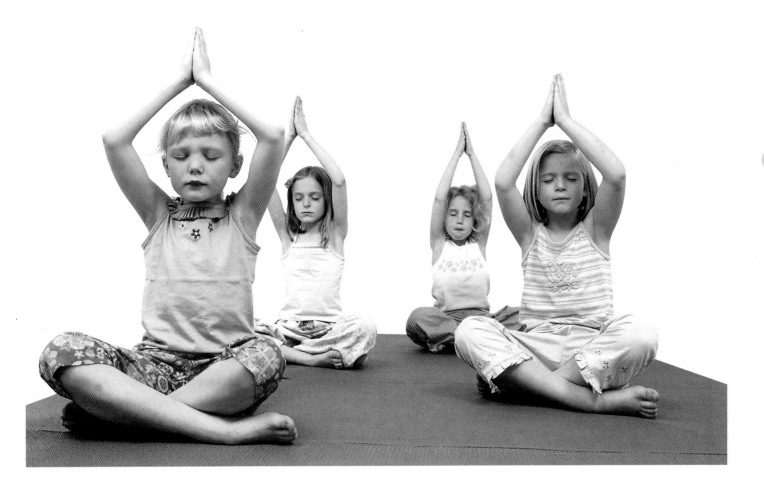

the breath as a bridge

The breath acts as a bridge between the mind and the body. You can see this in action by synchronizing simple stretches with your breathing patterns. Notice how the ebb and flow of your breath soothes your mind and helps your body to stretch.

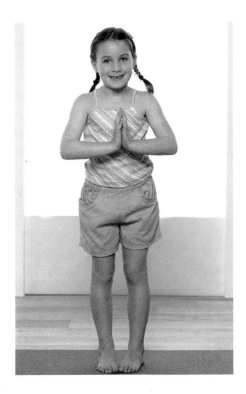

◁ The taller and straighter you stand, the better you breathe and the better you feel.

Your Invisible Friend
Who has seen the wind?
Neither you nor I,
But when the trees bow down
    their heads
The wind is passing by.

This poem illustrates that by seeing what the wind touches, we know it is there, even though we cannot see the wind itself. The same goes for our breath. If you blow a feather into the air, puff out a candle or watch your

△ Breathing slowly and deeply through your nose as you stretch your arms is a wonderfully empowering gesture that says "I am me!".

breath condense on a frosty day, you will see your breath at work. You can find "where" your breath is by using your hands. To do this, lie on your back, with your feet flat on the floor and your knees bent. Place both your hands, palms down, on your tummy. Position your hands so that they are covering your tummy button. Now feel the rise and fall of your breath.

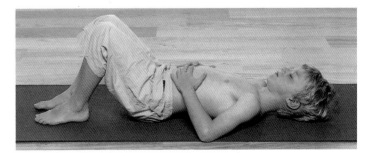

△ Tummy breathing is simply breathing with your hands on your tummy. Notice how your fingers gently separate as you breathe in and come together again as you breathe out.

Getting into the spirit

Yoga teaches us that we are more than just a collection of muscles and bones, and that we possess an inner spirit or soul. In many developed cultures, it is the appearance of the physical body that is championed and not what we are like on the inside. Not surprisingly, many people question whether the body does have a soul. However, the committed yogi would not only confirm its presence but would add that the soul is *the* essential element of our make-up.

our secret self

In yoga philosophy, the physical body is considered to be a vehicle for the soul on its journey towards truth and enlightenment. The soul represents man's true nature and identity. It is an inner world that lies not in the body's external casing but in the deeper *anandamaya kosha*, also known as the bliss sheath. Like a hidden jewel, the soul is always there for us to discover. It is always with us, just as the sun is always in the sky even though it may be hidden behind a bank of rain cloud.

reaching the soul

The regular practice of yoga can take us to this special internal place, so that we can experience the real us. Beginning to practise yoga asanas for physical reasons, to improve agility and strength or to ease a specific complaint such as backache, is the logical place to start. This gives us visible results and begins to break down our physical shell. As our awareness of our physical body grows, so too does our emotional sensitivity. We begin to experience things differently, and very soon it dawns on us that not only does yoga meet our initial expectations, but it gives us an extra something too.

"A man travels the world in search of the answers and comes home to find them."

showing your true colours

Yoga is a process of self-discovery, an unpeeling and unravelling, a working down through the layers until we reach our core. To begin with we may only glimpse the tranquillity of this inner sanctum, but over time, we may notice a subtle change in our approach to life. We feel more content with what we have got, rather than dissatisfied with what we don't have. We find that we have become more philosophical, more accepting of life's ups and downs, and less bothered by the little problems. This subtle, gradual evolution helps us to marvel at the spectacle of life rather than be overawed by its complexity.

less is more

For children, getting spiritual is about learning to tap into this inner joy. Yoga encourages us to use our natural, inner resources, and with guidance you will see that you have all you need to be happy within yourself.

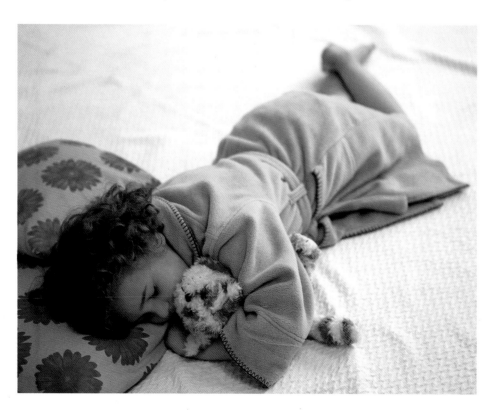

◁ Home is where the heart is. The security of a happy home environment makes for sweet dreams.

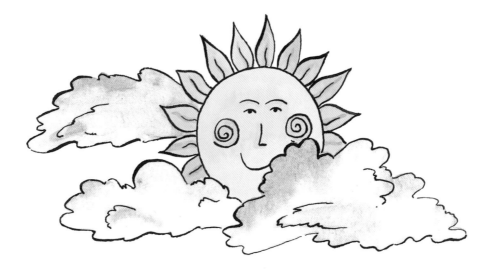

▷ Yoga philosophy states that we are all naturally sunny by nature. Simply blow away the clouds and see that the sun is still there, shining away as brightly as ever.

◁ Get your heads together! Group bonding helps you to enjoy the people you are close to, and to appreciate that life is all about giving and receiving love.

▽ Nothing beats the familiar feeling of a big hug from your favourite bear.

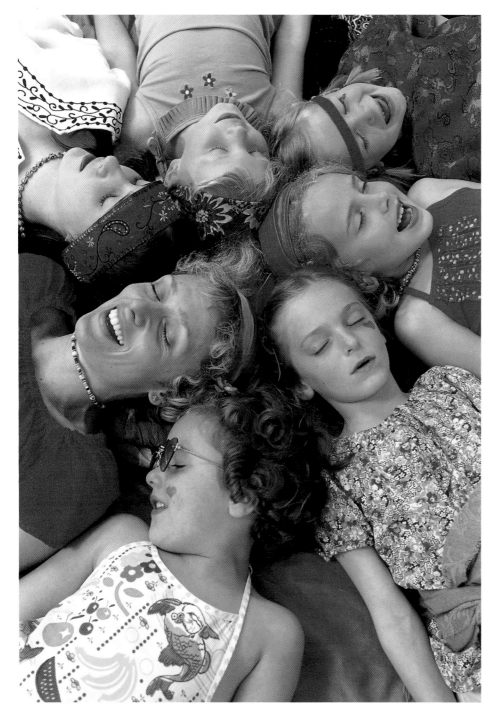

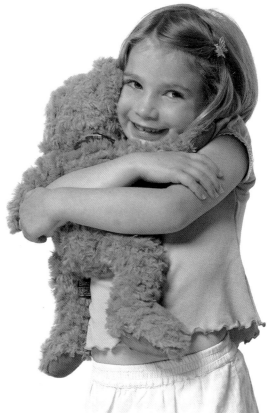

Finding the wizard within

All children can be encouraged to believe in themselves and to locate their inner strengths or powers. They only need to be shown how.

positive atttitudes

One aspect of yoga has to do with our actions. It means acting so that all of our attention is directed toward the activity to which we are engaged. This starts at home as we practise the physical aspects of yoga, and can then be applied to daily life.

Patanjali, author of the classic text *Yoga Sutras*, outlined a set of guidelines for living. These comprise *yamas*, which help us to check our behaviour, and *niyamas*, which help to refine our attitudes. Together they teach us to act in a conscientious and attentive manner in all that we do, making the very best of ourselves.

yamas

Non-aggression, or *ahimsa*, is one of the principal *yamas*. This encourages us to avoid injury in yoga asanas by underlining the importance of being nice to our bodies.

Developing compassion for others and protecting the environment are also aspects of the non-aggression principle. Always try to help others who are less fortunate than yourself, and take your litter home with you.

The honesty *yama*, known as *satya*, is about not trying to be what you are not. It asks us to know our strengths and weaknesses and to be proud of who and what we are.

Openness, known as *asteya*, teaches us to be flexible and open to change, allowing time for postures, like everyday situations, to evolve rather

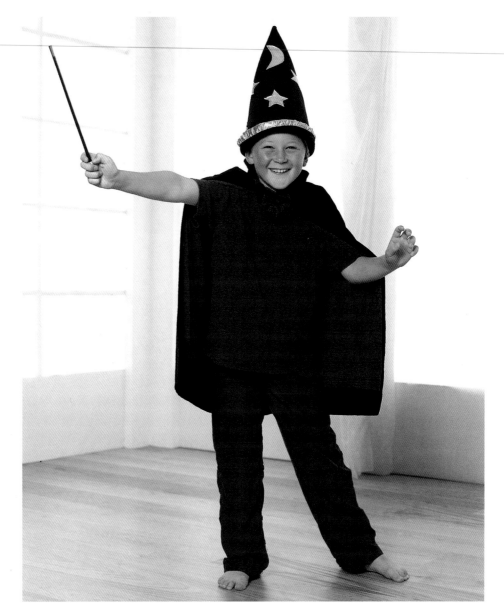

than trying to control them. *Asteya* literally means "to not steal", and it teaches us not to take advantage of others or to be jealous of what they have. It tells us to think about what we *have* got instead, and to nurture contentment within ourselves.

niyamas

Cleanliness, or *sauca*, is about living healthily and taking pride in our appearance. One way you could do this is to keep your bedroom tidy.

△ All of us have magical powers within ourselves, and with a bit of help from yoga we learn how to unleash them.

Contentment, known as *samtosa*, is about doing what we do because we enjoy it and not because other people are doing it.

Enthusiasm, known as *tapas*, literally means "heat". This is about keeping our passion for life alive: making the best of ourselves, putting in the effort and really going for it.

energy chakras

In yoga philosophy the chakras are invisible centres of spiritual and physical energy located in the body. They reflect our emotional state, and can affect our behaviour and attitudes. There are seven main chakras:

• Root or base (1) Feeling grounded and safe; the survival instinct
• Sacrum (2) Feelings about friends and family, social skills, and the ability to enjoy ourselves
• Solar plexus (3) Self-belief and enthusiasm for life
• Heart (4) Being open-hearted and joyful
• Throat (5) Communication
• Third eye (6) Clear thinking
• Crown (7) Wisdom and spirituality

Many yogis believe that learning to balance our chakras can help to restore harmony to our lives. Think about these energy centres and use visual imagery to bring them alive. A traditional image is the lotus flower. The idea is that when the petals of the lotus flower are closed, the chakra is closed too. Encouraging the petals to open and to be filled with a warm light is the way to bring back life and energy to the chakra. Try making up your own positive images that are relevant to you and your feelings.

Using visual imagery in this way can give all children a sense of the power of awareness. Don't be afraid to talk about your emotions. Ask yourself "where" in the body you feel sad or hurt. Describe and direct a visual image at the relevant chakra to help soothe emotional problems. Remember that a physical problem is often a sign of an underlying emotional imbalance.

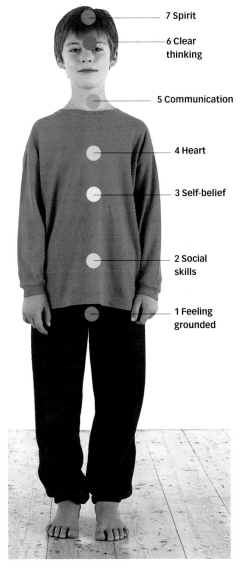

7 Spirit
6 Clear thinking
5 Communication
4 Heart
3 Self-belief
2 Social skills
1 Feeling grounded

open your heart

Rounded shoulders may mean that the heart chakra is closed. The heart chakra represents love for ourselves, for others and for life in general. Encourage open-heartedness and boost self-esteem by using upper body stretches that emphasize the meridians to the heart. Finger, arm and shoulder stretches are all good for this. Suitable stretches are found in the Lion, Fish and Camel poses.

▷ Sitting in Little Buddha pose keeps you grounded but helps your mind to think clearly.

introduction

◁ The seven chakras are located along our spine. Awareness of these special energy centres can enhance emotional well-being.

You could also visualize rays of warm sunlight flooding into the body in Little Buddha pose.

standing strong and still

The inability to concentrate or sit still can suggest a lack of grounding. Feeling able to stand on our own feet relates to our root chakra. Strong poses such as Warrior or Tree develop conviction, and make us feel anchored to life. Visualize a strong, majestic tree and feel its roots anchored deep in the earth. Try Little Buddha pose to feel grounded but still.

shout it out!

Shyness and the fear of speaking up relates to the throat chakra. Use sound to encourage self-expression and build confidence. Try Lion roar and Humming Bee Breath. Stretches that open up the chest, such as Cobra and Camel, may help too.

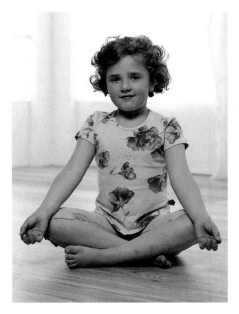

Let's warm up!

Warming up with gentle limbering exercises is essential preparation for your yoga practice. Spending just 5 or 10 minutes on these fun and simple exercises before you start your session will help to warm up cold muscles, focus your mind and get you in the mood. Preparing your body in this way is important as it will help you to avoid injury.

Keep the movements small to start with, working up from your feet and legs to your hands, wrists and arms, neck and head. Then move on to the body warm-ups and partner work.

getting started

- Choose a warm, light room in a quiet part of the house. Make sure the television is switched off!
- Wait a good hour or two after a meal before you start your yoga session.
- Practise on a rug or carpet or your own yoga mats if you have them.
- Wear loose, comfortable clothes.
- Have some soft cushions handy and, for younger children, a few soft toys as props.
- Light some candles or mild incense to set the mood.
- Play some relaxing music for the quiet time session.
- Plan for a 15 minute session and build it up gradually to 30 minutes as you become used to it. Use your body language and energy levels as your guide, and learn to recognize when enough is enough.
- Aim to make your yoga positive not perfect. Have fun!

planning a yoga session

- Do some of the warm-up exercises before you start.
- Practise nasal breathing.
- Come in and out of postures gently and thoughtfully – asana means "comfortable seat", and you should always feel at ease in the poses you do.
- Encourage self-expression by accompanying animal poses with sound: roar like a lion! bark like a dog!
- Balance the body by doing postures on both sides of the body.
- Erase the last posture by following it with a counter pose. For example, follow a forward bend with a backward bend, and lie down to rest after a series of strong standing poses.
- Poses that twist the spine are best done after you have stretched the back forwards, as in the Rag Doll pose (standing forward bend).

- Think about linking breath to movement and, as a general rule, breathe in when you stretch up or back and out when you fold forwards or down (the Sunshine Stretch is a good example of this).
- Sequence your session with asanas, games, breathing exercises and quiet time, and always end a session with at least 5–10 minutes in relaxation, or longer if you like.
- Keep a yoga diary using stick men to show the postures you have done. Record feelings and sensations and talk about which parts of the session you enjoyed the most.

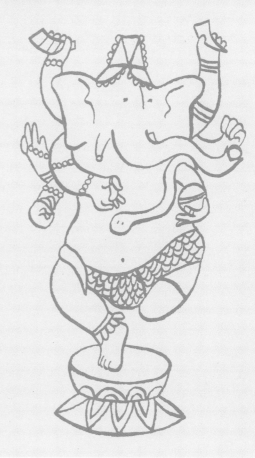

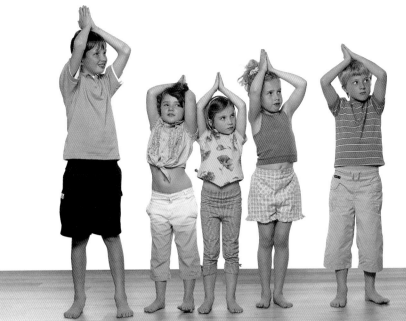

◁ **Spinning top** Make a pointy hat by holding your hands together above your head. Now draw an invisible circle with your pointy hat to wake up your waist.

▷ **Draw circles** Use your feet, your hands and your hips to draw circles in the air. Make circles of different sizes; the slower you can make them the better. If there are a few of you, you may want to hold hands to stop yourselves falling over!

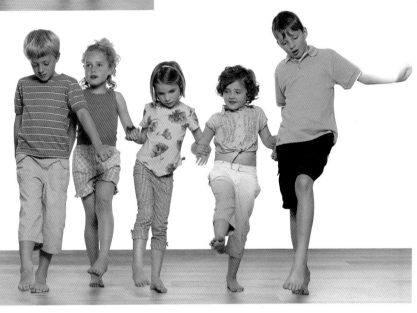

◁ **Windmill arms** Gently circle your arms like the sails of a windmill. Breathe in as you stretch up your arms, and breathe out as your arms come back down to your lap.

▷ **Shoulder shrugs** Squeeze your shoulders up to your ears as you breathe in, and round behind you and down again as you breathe out. Notice how long your neck feels now.

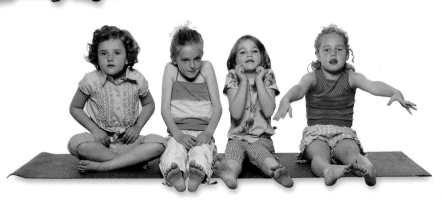

▷

Rocking the baby

This warm up gives a strong stretch to your hips and buttocks. Imagine your lower leg is a little baby that you are gently rocking to sleep in your arms. Cradle your lower leg as you would a sleeping child and rock from side to side, breathing deeply. Lift your foot to kiss the baby's forehead.

1 Sitting on your bottom, lift up your right leg and gently bend your knee. Draw your right foot in towards your tummy button, cradling your ankle in your hand.

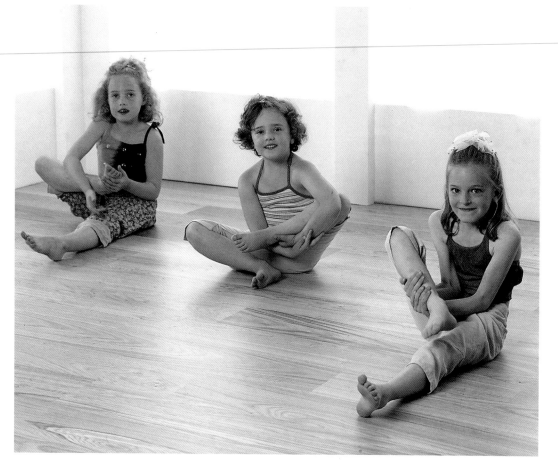

2 Hug your knee and lower leg with your arms and gently rock your baby from side to side. Finish off with a little kiss on your baby's forehead as you lift your foot towards your face.

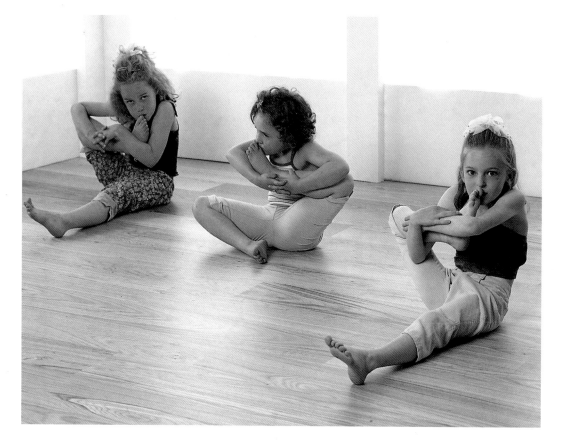

Cat, dog, snake and mouse

Do as many rounds of this flowing animal warm-up sequence as you like. It wakes up your back, stretches your legs and strengthens your arms, wrists and hands. You can do the sequence on your own but it is much more fun to do it in pairs. Let each part merge into the next and don't forget to breathe!

1 Kneel on the floor in Cat pose, with your shoulders over your hands and your claws (your fingers) spread wide. Rub noses with your cat friend and breathe in deeply.

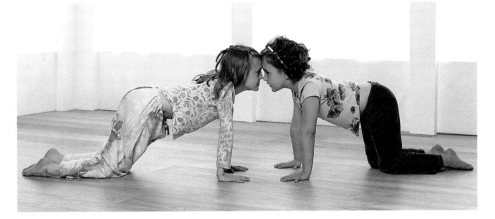

2 As you breathe out, curl your toes under and lift your knees and bottom upwards, letting your head hang forward and down. Let your heels sink into the floor as you imagine you are a dog doing his morning stretch. Take a few more breaths.

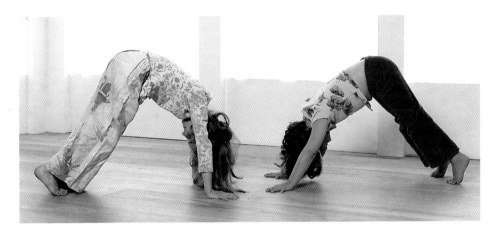

3 As you take your next breath in, roll over your toes and let your hips and tummy drop to the floor. Point your toes behind you, stick out your tongue and hiss like a snake. Keep breathing steadily.

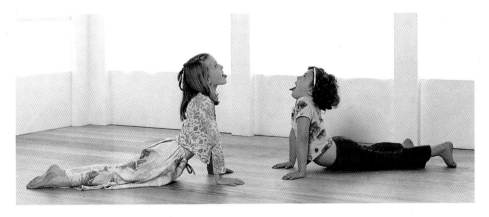

4 Lift your bottom up as you breathe out and sit back on your heels with your forehead on the floor. Rest like a quiet little mouse. Then lift your bottom up to come back to Cat pose, and start all over again.

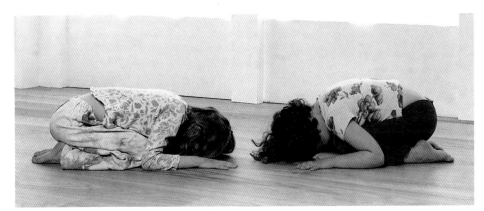

▷

Partner work

Doing limbering exercises and yoga postures in twos gives you double the fun. You can make your stretches deeper when you have someone to help you. Working together makes you more considerate and helps you to develop responsibility for your partner. Talk to each other as you do these exercises to help each other get the most out of each movement.

At a spiritual level, partner work builds connectedness and reinforces the concept of yoga – to unite. It is a wonderful way to bond relationships and to promote the idea of sharing.

◁ **Table top** Stand facing each other and place your palms on each other's shoulders. Hold on gently but firmly and then step away from each other until the crowns of your heads come together. Keep hold of your partner's shoulders and stretch your bottom back, so that your back flattens. Breathe deeply then walk your feet in towards each other and relax.

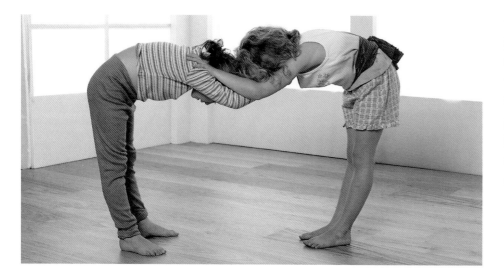

▷ **Rainbow** In this pose the sides of your bodies create the arc of a beautiful rainbow. Kneel down about 1m/3ft away from each other, with your bottoms lifted off your heels. Extend your outside legs, and rest your inside hands on the floor between you for support. Breathe in and, as you breathe out, bring your outside arms up and put your hands together to give a lovely stretch to the upper side of your body. Picture a rainbow filling you with its vibrant light. Release and change sides.

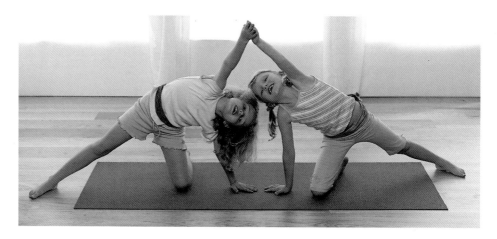

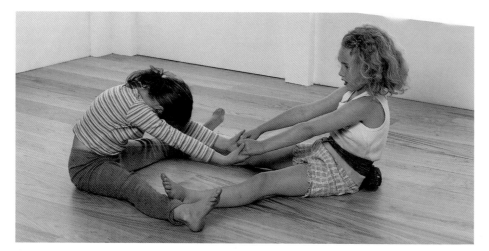

◁ **Seesaw** Sit opposite each other with your legs outstretched. One of you needs to place the balls of your feet against the inside of your partner's shins. Reach forward and take her hands. Gently pull her forwards towards you so that she gets a lovely stretch in her back and the backs of her legs. Release and swap.

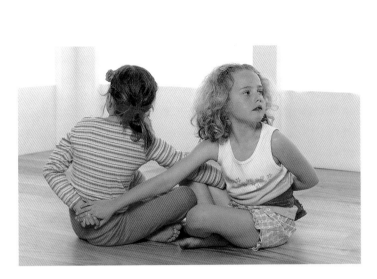

△ **Figure of eight** Sit opposite your partner with crossed legs and your knees touching. Reach your right arm forward and down towards your partner's right arm. Fold your left arm behind you and reach round to grasp your partner's right hand. Breathe steadily and deeply and on each out-breath, gently pull your partner's left hand towards you. Hold for a few long breaths, then change arms.

△ **Washing windows** Kneel opposite each other, raise your arms and press your palms together. Imagine you have a sheet of glass between you. Here one of you guides the other's hands as you wash the window, and one of you will let yourself be guided. Draw big circles, reaching as high up and as far to the sides and down towards your knees as you can. Keep the hands together as you make the circles.

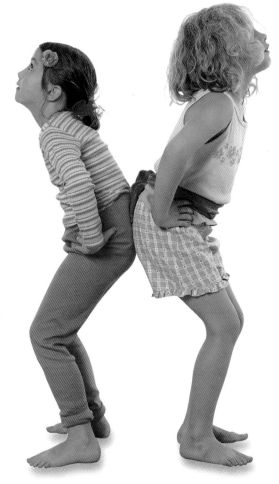

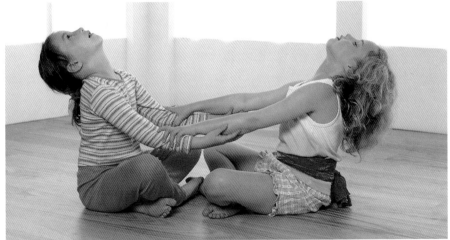

△ **The fountain** Sit cross-legged on the floor. Hold each other's lower arms. Breathe in and, as you breathe out, lean back and allow your partner to support your body. Do this one at a time to begin with, then do it both together.

◁ **Chair** Stand with your backs to each other, feet apart. Squat down until your bottoms touch, and put your hands on your hips. Breathe deeply. When your legs begin to ache, imagine energy flowing between you so that you can hold the pose for a few more breaths. Release and relax.

did you know that...

Ligaments and muscles need to be stretched gradually and naturally without hurry or forcing. This is especially true during childhood, when the muscles are still growing. This is what makes warm-up exercises so important.

Sunshine stretch

This sequence was designed as a greeting to the sun god, which in Hindu mythology is worshipped as a symbol of health and immortality.

The Sunshine Stretch limbers up and energizes the whole body, particularly the back, making it flexible and strong. It also clears your mind, puts a smile on your face and makes you ready for the day ahead.

Stand in front of a window for this sequence, particularly if the sun is shining, or stand opposite a friend. Breathing deeply will help each part of the sequence flow into the next. As a general rule, you breathe in as you stretch up or backwards and breathe out when you bend forwards.

"Truly, a flexible back makes for a long life." CHINESE PROVERB

1 Stand in Mountain pose, or *tadasana*, looking straight in front of you – facing your partner or a window – with your legs straight and your feet together. Hold your hands in Namaste, or prayer position. Breathe deeply and imagine a cord from the crown of your head, gently drawing you upwards while your feet remain firmly grounded.

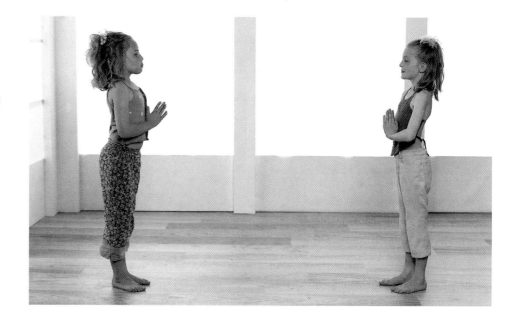

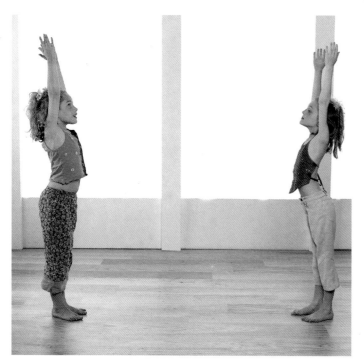

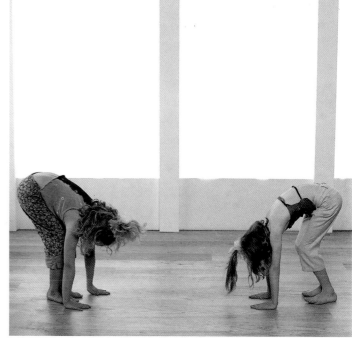

2 Stretch your arms up high above your head as you breathe in. Bring your palms together and hold for a few seconds.

3 Now exhale and fold forwards, bending your knees, and bring your hands to the ground in front of you, keeping your palms flat.

a summary of the movements

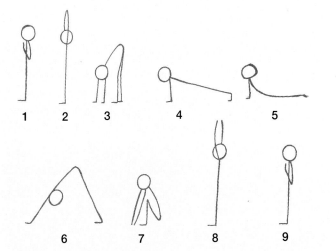

1 2 3 4 5

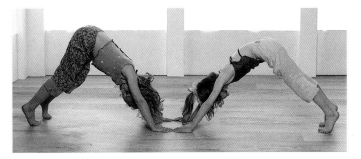

6 7 8 9

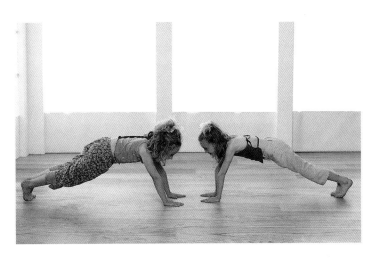

4 Step one leg back as far as you can, and then the other. Push back through your heels, keeping your legs straight. Imagine that your whole body feels like a stiff, strong plank of wood.

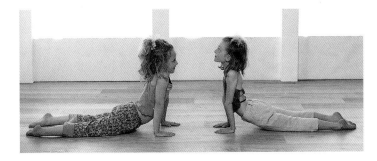

5 Lower your legs to the floor, drop your hips forwards and arch your back as you breathe out. Keep your head up. This is Cobra pose.

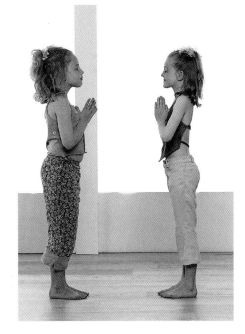

6 Breathe in and, as you breathe out, tuck your toes under and lift your bottom up into Dog pose. Hold here for a few breaths. Try to sink your heels into the floor and straighten your legs.

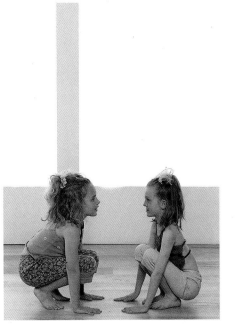

7 As you breathe out, bend your knees and look forwards so that you are facing each other. Then jump both feet forwards towards your hands and squat down.

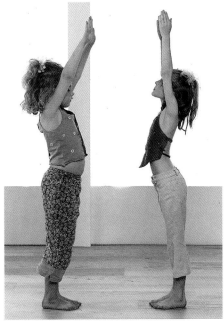

8 Now straighten your legs and lift your arms up high above your head with palms together. Breathe in deeply. Stretch upwards to make yourself grow as tall as you can. Hold for a few breaths.

9 Breathe out and bring your hands into Namaste, or prayer position, in front of you. This completes the Sunshine Stretch. Repeat as many times as you like until your whole body feels warm and alive.

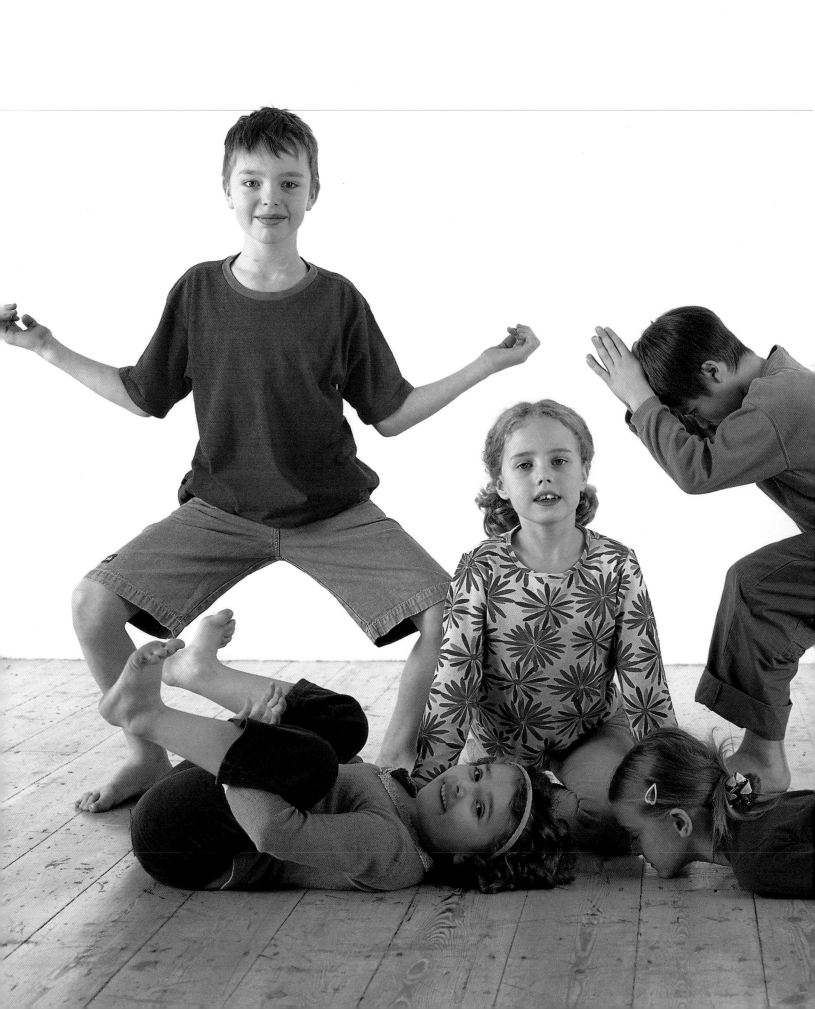

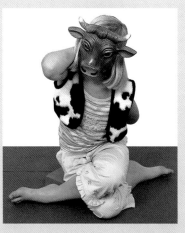

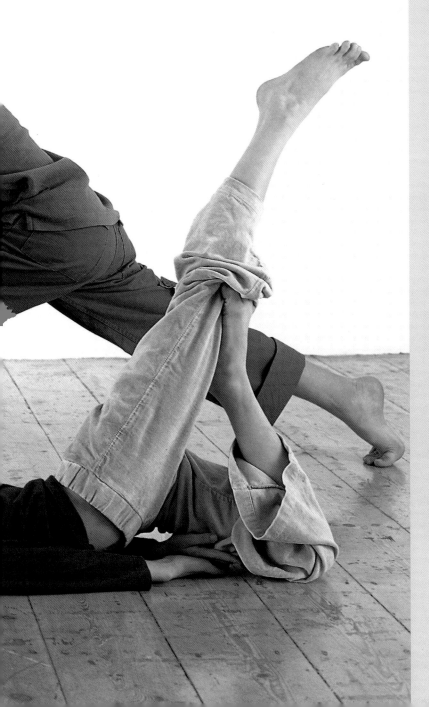

animal
parade

This section allows you to have some fun

as you come face to face with a parade

of animals of all shapes and sizes. These

expressive poses show children how to

imitate the instinctive behaviour and

movements of their favourite creatures,

birds and insects, and lets them assume the

characteristics of each. Feel the power and

pride of the roaring lion or soaring eagle,

the quiet serenity of a fluttering butterfly,

the suppleness of a slithering snake and the

joyful agility of a leaping frog.

Lion

Lion pose – **Simhasana**
Roaring lion – **Simhagarjanasana**

The lion is known as the king of beasts. He sleeps in the heat of the day and hunts by night, when it is cooler and his energy levels are at their highest. This is a very simple pose that all children love, and it is easy enough for even the very young or those who are new to yoga. It is lots of fun, and things can get quite noisy when everybody starts to roar!

benefits

Lion pose will energize the body and mind. It builds self-confidence and improves communication skills. In addition, it dispels nerves and physical tension in the face, and helps to allay sore throats and problems with the eyes, ears, nose and mouth. It also clears your mind, makes you smile and gets you ready to start the day.

when to do the pose

This is a good pose for when energy levels need a boost. It can also be very helpful before an important event that may be making you feel anxious and a little apprehensive. Because it is so easy to do, it is suitable for children of all ages. It is a fun way to start a yoga session, especially if the children can make a nice loud roar.

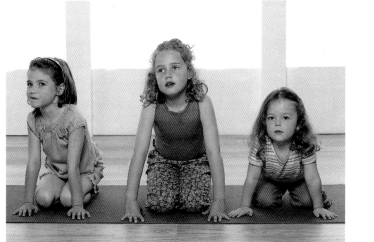

a summary of the movements

1

2

1 First, bend your knees and sit on your heels with your hands on the floor in front of you. Then rest your hands – which are now your paws – gently on your lap. Sit quietly, breathing gently.

2 Breathe in steadily and sit forwards on your knees, with your hands and arms out in front of you. Roarrrrr! Look upwards and stick out your tongue. Now sit back on your heels and roar in this way twice more to make yourself feel powerful but calm.

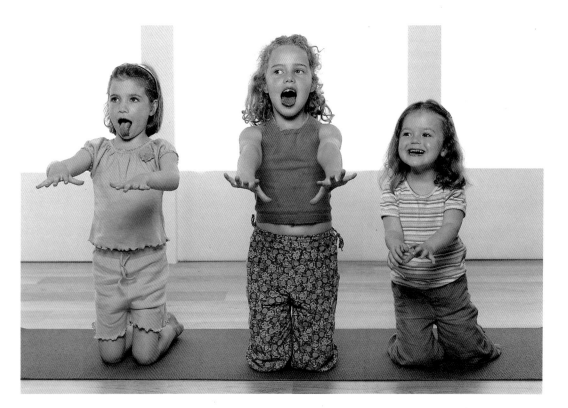

Dog

Adho mukha svanasana

Domestic dogs have been man's best friend for thousands of years. The Downward Facing Dog is a classic pose that imitates the stretch that dogs do when they wake up. It combines an instinctive grace with a lovely elongation of the whole back.

benefits

This pose will give you energy. It also stretches the back from the tailbone to the top of the neck, and strengthens wrists, hands, arms and shoulders. It brings fresh blood to the head and helps to release stiffness in the neck.

when to do the pose

Do this gentle stretching pose when you get out of bed in the morning, or as part of your warm-up sequence before a yoga session. It is particularly good as preparation for the Sunshine Stretch.

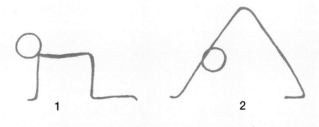

▽ Downward Facing Dog at full stretch.

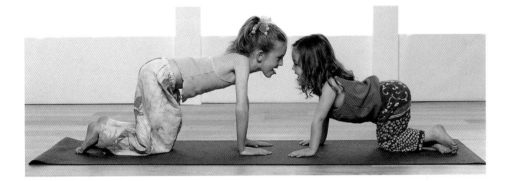

1 ◁ Rest in cat pose on all fours. Your knees should be under your hips and your hands under your shoulders. Spread your fingers wide and spread your body weight evenly into each hand. Curl your toes under.

2 ▽ Breathe in, and as you breathe out, lift your knees off the floor and push your bottom upwards. Keep the legs a little bent to begin with and push your chest gently back towards your thighs. Walk your heels up and down a few times. Then try to release both heels to the floor, straightening your legs as much as you can. Imagine someone lifting you up by your tailbone so that your body resembles the two sides of a capital "A". Look back towards your tailbone, allowing your head to feel really heavy. Breathe deeply. To come out of the pose, drop to your knees and sit back on your heels, with your forehead on the floor. Relax.

a summary of the movements

1

2

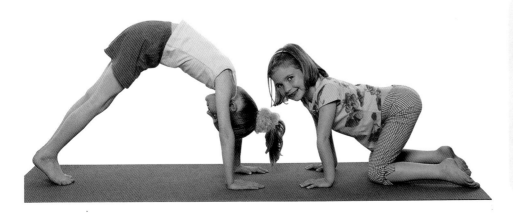

variation

Now try the Upward Facing Dog, which turns the pose into a back bend. From Downward Facing Dog, bend your knees and rest them on the floor. Push your hips forwards, but keep them off the floor. Push into your hands, lift your chest and look up as you gently arch your back.

Cobra

Bhujangasana

In this strong, energizing back bend, let your legs feel really heavy and keep them still so that the top half of your body can rear up strongly, like a cobra poised to strike. Feel free to hiss as loudly as you like.

benefits
Cobra pose keeps the spine supple and healthy, and tones the nerves, improving communication between the brain and the body. It also helps to stimulate the appetite.

when to do the pose
Practise Cobra when you are feeling floppy and in need of an energy boost. It is also good for when you want to feel strong and powerful.

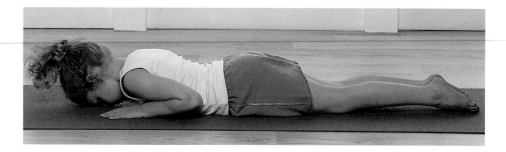

1 Lie on the floor with your forehead touching the ground. Tuck your elbows in at your sides and place the palms of your hands under your shoulders. Concentrate on keeping your legs and hips heavy. Push your feet into the floor.

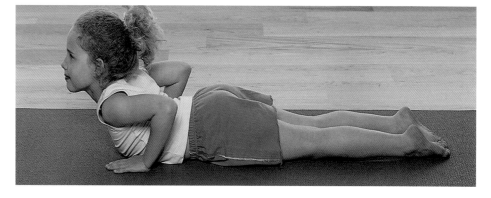

2 Breathe in deeply and, as you do so, slowly lift your head off the ground. Begin to look upwards as you push your hands into the floor. Keep your legs out straight behind you, with your toes pointed and your feet pushed into the floor.

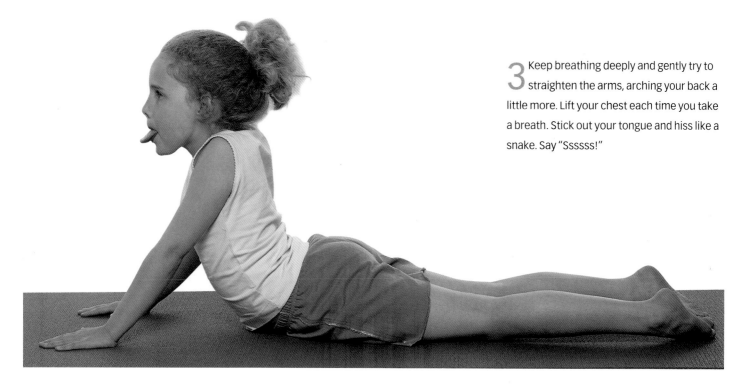

3 Keep breathing deeply and gently try to straighten the arms, arching your back a little more. Lift your chest each time you take a breath. Stick out your tongue and hiss like a snake. Say "Sssssss!"

4 If you fancy scratching your head with your tail, simply widen your knees and arch your back a little more as you raise your feet towards your head. Gently lie down again and curl yourself up in Child's pose, sitting on your heels and resting your forehead on the floor in front of you, with your arms lying relaxed by your sides. This is a counter pose to "unsnake" your back.

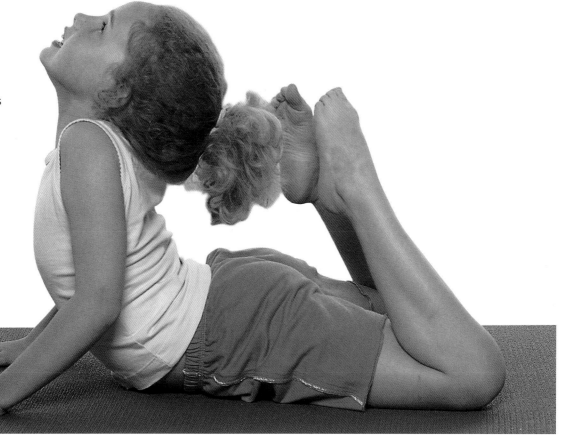

a summary of the movements

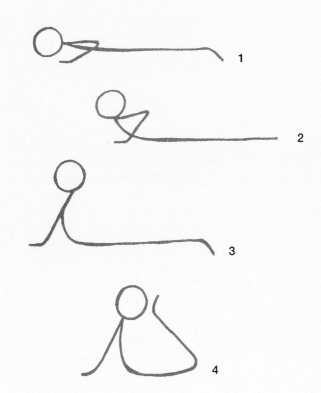

1

2

3

4

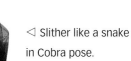 Slither like a snake in Cobra pose.

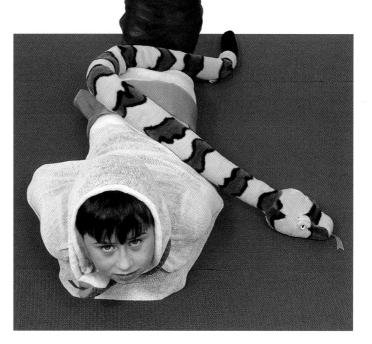

Eagle

Garudasana

One minute the golden eagle can be standing motionless, high on a mountain top, scanning the landscape. The next minute he can summon all his energy, stretch out his enormous wing span and plunge through the air at speed in the search for prey. Eagle pose is a standing balance that mimics the poise and strength of the golden eagle.

benefits

Eagle pose is very good for nurturing determination and inner conviction. It also helps you to concentrate and makes your legs feel really strong.

when to do the pose

This is a good movement for when you are feeling uptight or unsure, and need to find some inner strength.

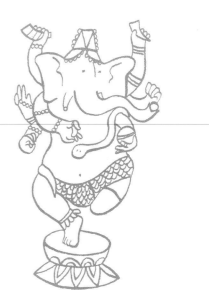

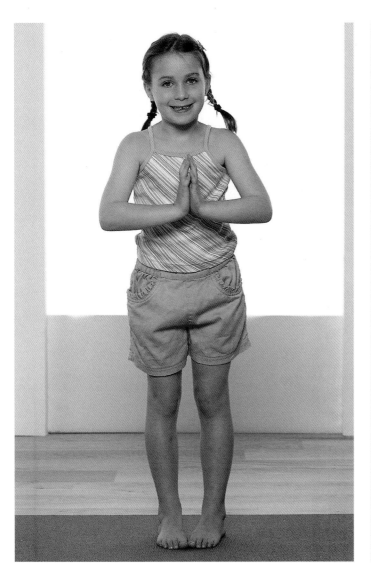

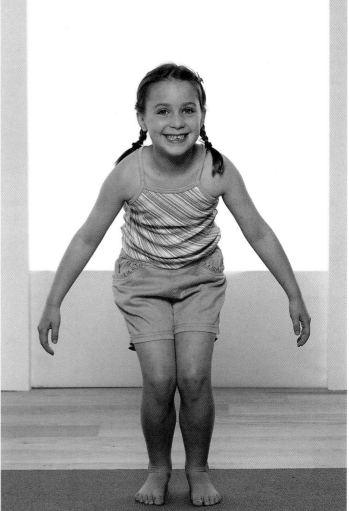

1 Stand in Mountain pose, or *tadasana*, looking straight in front of you with your legs straight and your feet together. Put your hands in prayer position, or Namaste. Visualize a beautiful golden eagle perched high on the peak of a mountain, looking down majestically on to the valley below. Steady your breath.

2 As you breathe out, bend your knees and spread your arms out to your sides like a pair of wings. Feel yourself firmly rooted in the floor. You are the eagle high on the mountain peak.

a summary of the movements

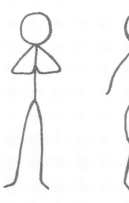 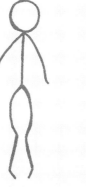 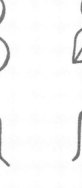

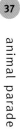

1   **2**   **3**   **4**

4 ▽ Make a soft fist with your right hand and place it under your chin. Support your elbow with your left palm. Breathe steadily for a few moments. Release the pose, shake out your arms and legs, and repeat on the other side.

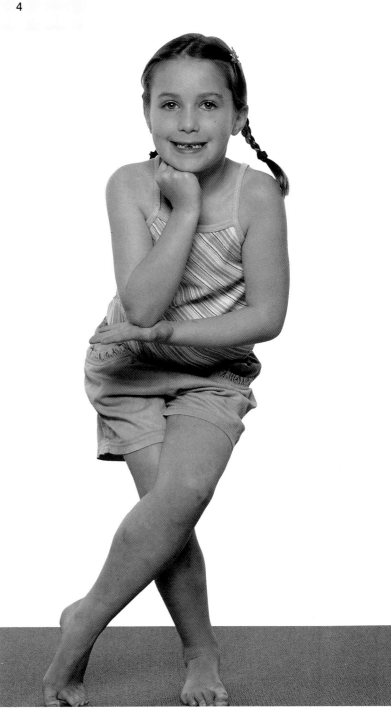

3 Keeping both of your knees bent, cross your left leg over your right so that the ball of your left foot makes contact with the floor just to the side of your right foot.

Fish

Matsyasana

In Hindu mythology the God Vishnu turned himself into a fish, or *matsya*, to save the world from the flood. Fish pose is a gentle yet powerful back bend in which the raised chest mimics the rounded back of a fish. In the pose you lie on the floor with your knees bent and your back arched.

benefits

Fish encourages deep breathing and can give relief to mild symptoms of asthma and bronchitis. The graceful arching of the back opens up the chest, keeping the heart chakra open and releasing positive feelings of love and well-being.

when to do the pose

Use Fish to improve posture and chase away negative feelings. You can do it after Shoulder Stand, Candle or Dragonfly pose too. The very young may find this pose a bit too much for them. They can try Crocodile instead, which has many of the same benefits.

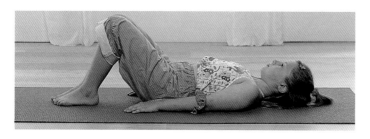

1 Lie on the floor with your knees bent, legs together and feet flat on the floor. Your arms should lay straight by your sides.

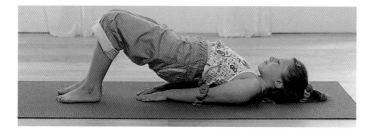

2 Breathe in and, keeping your knees bent, lift your bottom off the floor and slide your hands underneath. Bring your hands close together so that the fingers touch.

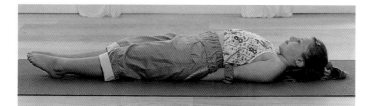

3 Lie down on your hands. Extend your legs and allow them to feel heavy. Let your breath become steady.

a summary of the movements

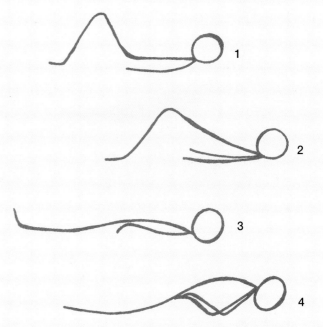

4 On a breath in, push up your chest, letting your back arch and the top of your head roll on to the floor. Push your elbows down. Take five deep breaths, then release to the floor, slide out your hands and hug your knees.

Frog

Malasana

Frogs are cold-blooded amphibians that start life without any limbs at all. They develop arms and legs as they grow older, and by the time they are adult frogs their legs are strong and very springy. This is a fun action pose that grows from a quiet squat into an explosive leap upwards into the air.

benefits

Frog is good for strengthening the upper and lower legs and making them more flexible. It also helps to tone the ankles and feet. It is a fantastic way to raise energy levels quickly if you are feeling tired but still have lots of things to get done.

when to do the pose

Leap like a frog when you feel tired and lethargic and want a quick boost of energy, or if you feel over-excited and need to let off some steam. Because this is quite a sudden, jerky movement, it should only be done after the warm-up exercises.

a summary of the movements

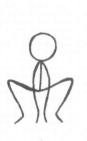
1

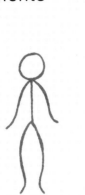
2

3

4

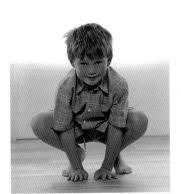

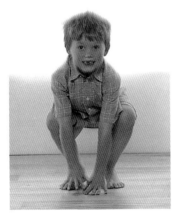

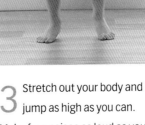

1 Crouch down on the floor with your knees wide and the palms of your hands flat on the floor in front of you. Breathe steadily and visualize your legs becoming strong like a frog's.

2 When you feel ready, push down into your hands and feet and spring upwards.

3 Stretch out your body and jump as high as you can. Make frog noises as loud as you can – "Grribbiid!"

4 Try to land on both feet as you come down from the jump. Crouch down again, ready to repeat the jump. Sit quietly for a few seconds when you have had enough jumping.

Crocodile

Makarasana

This playful posture will encourage self-expression and is fun to practise in a group. Look out for it later on in the book in the children's game called Snap and Snack.

benefits
Crocodile pose strengthens the back and gives you energy. If you find yourself in a bad mood, Crocodile can help release anger and aggression.

when to do the pose
When you feel low or cross, Crocodile helps you to get rid of negative feelings and will brighten your mood.

▽ The crocodile is a fierce fighter.

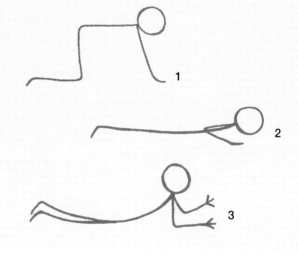

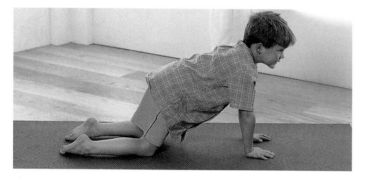

1 Kneel on the floor in Cat pose, with your shoulders over your hands and your fingers spread wide. Stretch out your legs behind you.

a summary of the movements

1

2

3

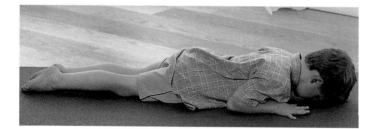

2 Lie down on the floor and bring your hands underneath your shoulders with your elbows tucked into your sides. Spread your fingers like claws. Make a heavy tail by bringing your legs together. Rest your forehead on the floor and visualize yourself as a crocodile.

3 As you breathe in, lift your legs and rear up your head. Keep swishing your tail from side to side to help you slither forwards and sideways. When you have had enough, curl up in Child's pose to release your back.

Crow

Kakasana

The black crow is the largest of the songbirds. He has strong feet and legs to enable him to move swiftly and purposefully on land, and broad wings that help him to soar powerfully in the air. In this pose your hands turn into the crow's feet and your back becomes his body. This pose requires strength, confidence and concentration. Imagine the beady eye of a crow to help you concentrate on the position.

benefits

Crow pose focuses the mind. It also strengthens the wrists, arms and upper body, and helps to develop physical balance and co-ordination.

when to do the pose

Do Crow when you feel apprehensive about something and your mind is jumpy. It will help you feel in control and will strengthen inner conviction.

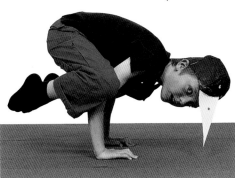

▽ Rising to the challenge in Crow pose.

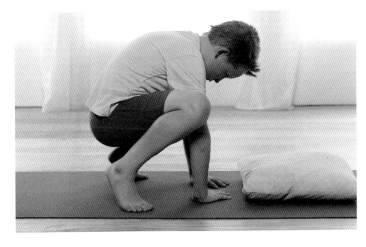

1 Place a cushion on the floor, and then squat down with your feet hip-width apart and the cushion in front of you. Place your palms on the floor with your fingers spread out and turned slightly inwards.

a summary of the movements

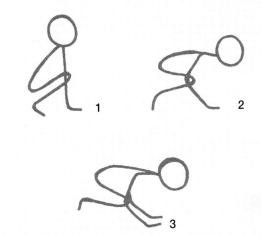

1

2

3

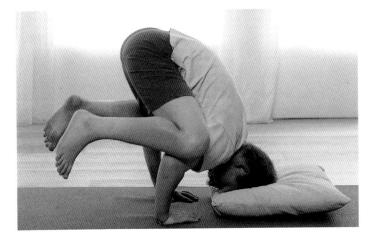

2 Press your upper arms against the inside of your knees. Start to rock forwards until you feel your body weight spreading on to your hands. Rock back to transfer the weight to your feet. Use the cushion for support and don't worry if you lose your balance, just keep trying.

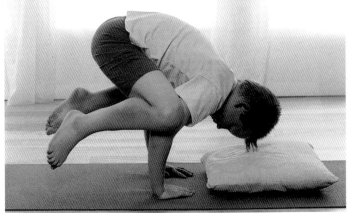

3 With practice you will be able to balance on your hands for longer and longer. Then bring your feet together to make your crow's tail. Hold for as long as you can and then lower your feet and release.

Blue whale

Setu bandhasana

The yogis called this Bridge pose because it makes your tummy look like a bridge. But being a big blue whale is more fun!

The blue whale is the largest living animal and even though it weighs as much as 15 elephants, it still manages to be graceful. Blue Whale pose is an energizing back bend. The lower part of the body makes the back of a big blue whale – imagine your navel is its blowhole. Start off from Dead Man pose, lying on the floor with the feet hip-width apart, the arms away from the body and the eyes closed.

benefits

Blue Whale pose is very good for strengthening the back and leg muscles, and it gives a nice stretch to the back of the neck. It helps to keep the spine supple and opens up the heart, chest and lungs.

when to do the pose

Practise Blue Whale pose when you need a little lift after something has upset you. Not only can this help to calm you down, it will also help to relieve backache.

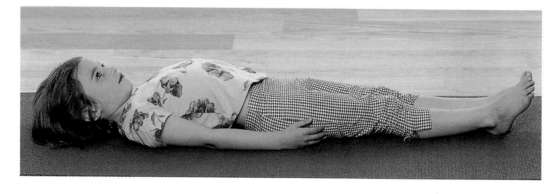

1 Lie down on your back in Dead Man pose. Rest your arms by your sides and steady your breathing.

2 Bend your knees so that your feet are flat on the floor, hip-width apart and a little away from your bottom. Keep your arms at your sides.

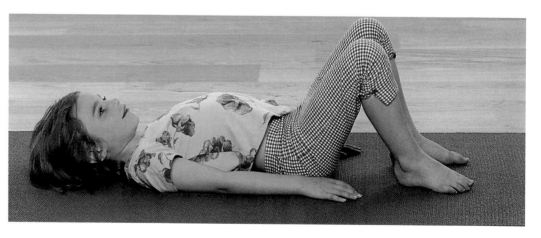

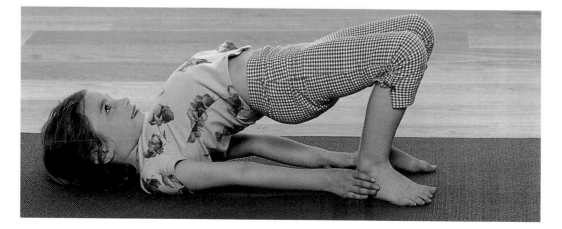

3 Breathe in and slowly peel your back off the ground. Breathe out and imagine you are spurting water out of your tummy button – just like the whale's blowhole.

a summary of the movements

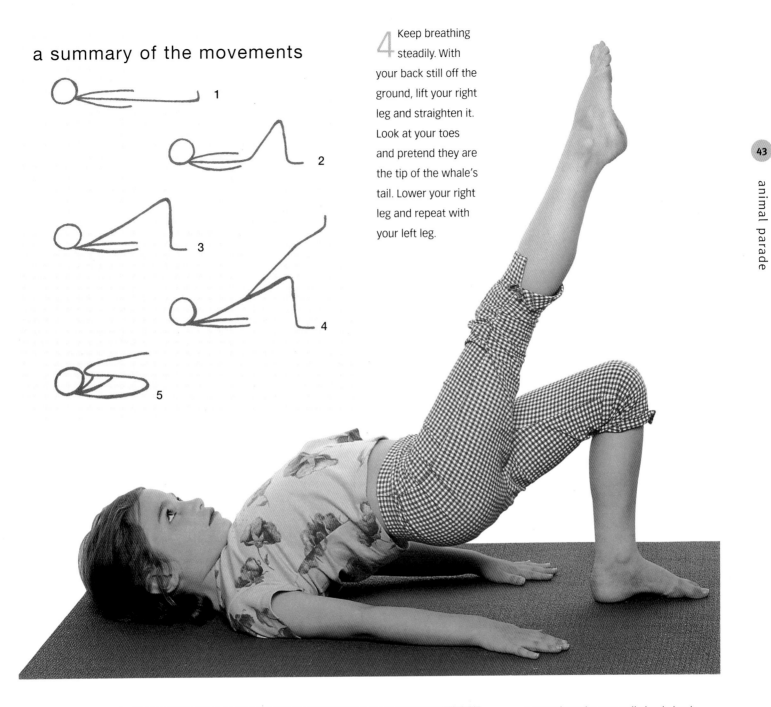

4 Keep breathing steadily. With your back still off the ground, lift your right leg and straighten it. Look at your toes and pretend they are the tip of the whale's tail. Lower your right leg and repeat with your left leg.

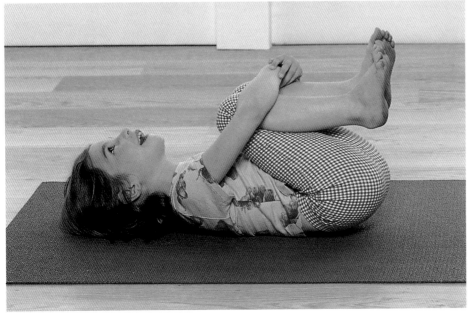

5 As you breathe out, roll slowly back down to the floor again and hug your knees to your chest like an upturned beetle. This is a counter pose to release your back.

Butterfly

Baddha konasana

The butterfly is a wonderful example of transformation. It starts its life as a humble caterpillar and evolves into a beautiful, winged creature. This simple seated pose will help your hips to become more flexible, allowing your spine to elongate. Try sitting on a cushion if you find it hard to sit up directly on the floor.

benefits

This will give your inner thighs a lovely gentle stretch, and will help to improve your posture when seated. It will also help you to feel grounded.

when to do the pose

Practise Butterfly in preparation for Little Buddha pose and to relax your legs after Rocking the Baby, as part of your warm-up sequence.

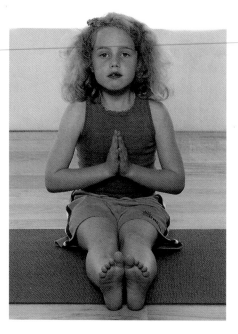

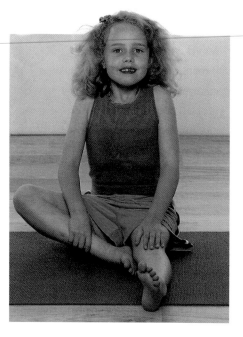

1 Sit on the floor with both of your legs outstretched in front of you and your feet together. Hold your hands in prayer position, or Namaste, and look straight ahead.

2 Bend your right leg and bring the sole of the foot into the inside of your left thigh. Hold the position.

▽ Learning Butterfly pose will help you to sit up straight.

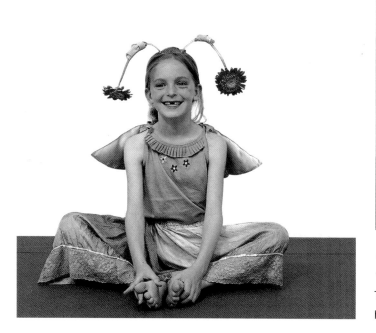

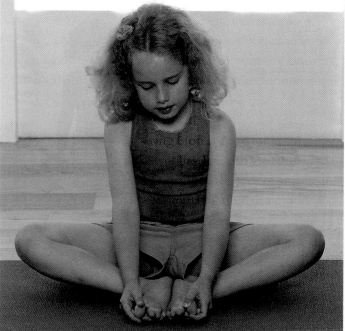

3 Then bring the left leg in so that the soles of your feet are together. You will now be able to feel a gentle stretch of your inner thighs. Try opening your feet with your hands like the covers of a book. This will help your knees to drop open a little more.

4 Then interlace your fingers and place them under the outer edges of your feet. Sit up tall, with your back nice and straight.

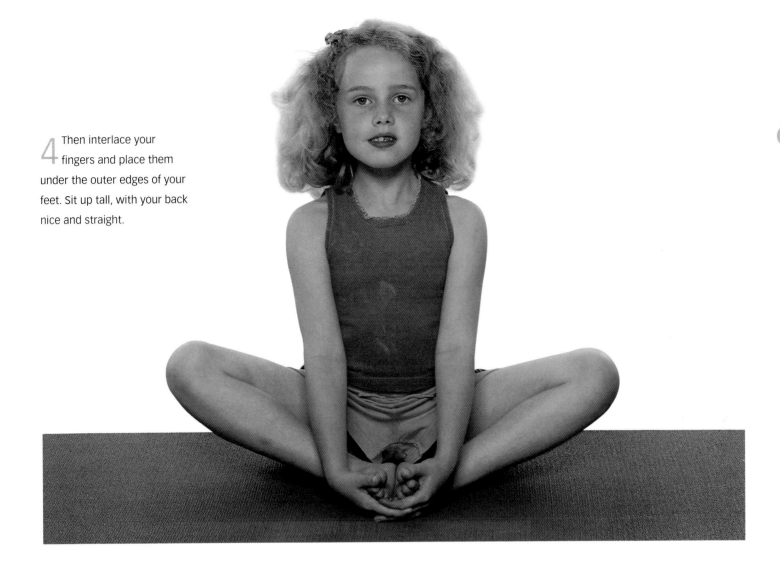

a summary of the movements

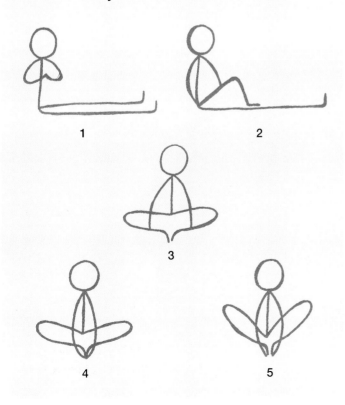

1

2

3

4

5

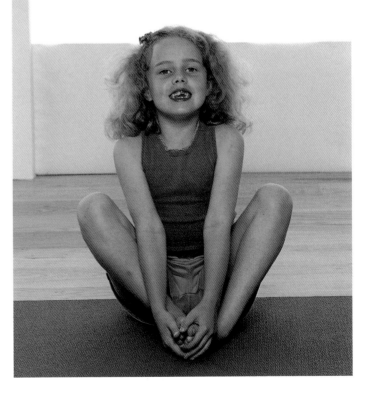

5 Gently lift and lower your knees as if you are a butterfly flapping its delicate, colourful wings. Relax.

Pigeon

Kapotasana

Homing pigeons have an in-built compass that allows them to navigate their way home, no matter how far they have flown.

benefits

Pigeon pose will give a deep, long stretch to your buttock muscles. The forward bending stage of this pose is particularly good at helping to calm an agitated mind.

when to do the pose

Pigeon energizes the body after a busy day or after a series of strong standing poses, such as Warrior and Triangle.

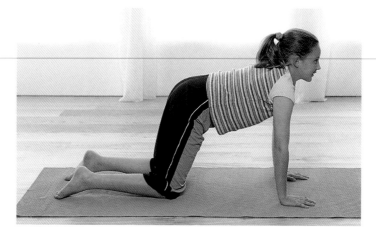

1 Get down on your hands and knees in Cat pose.

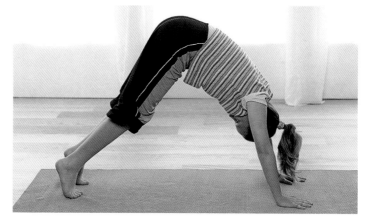

2 Now tuck under your toes, lift your knees and come into Dog pose. Take a moment to stretch out your legs.

3 Then lift your left leg upwards, bend the knee and lunge it through your hands.

a summary of the movements

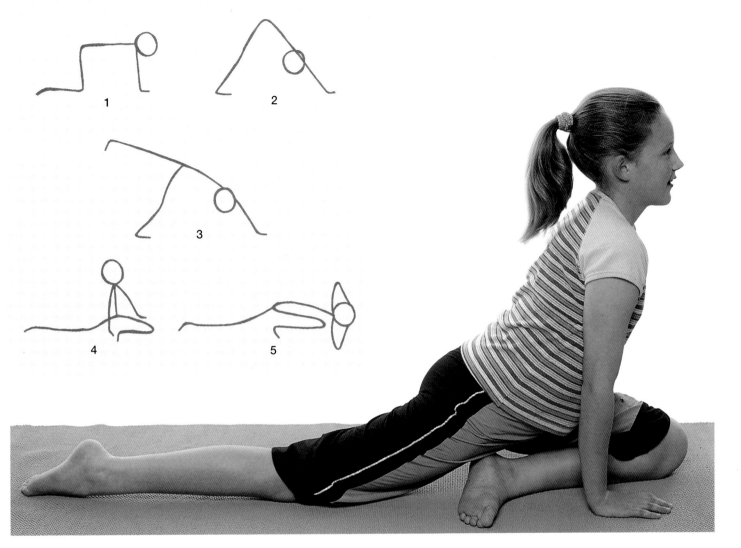

1 2 3 4 5

4 △ Place the knee on the floor and bring the heel to the right. Sit to the outside of your left knee. Let the back of your left thigh release on to the floor. Stretch out your right leg and prop yourself up with your hands.

5 ▽ Breathe steadily and, as you exhale, lean your chest forwards over your knee. Make a pillow with your hands and relax. Close your eyes for a few minutes. Release and rest in Child's pose, then change sides.

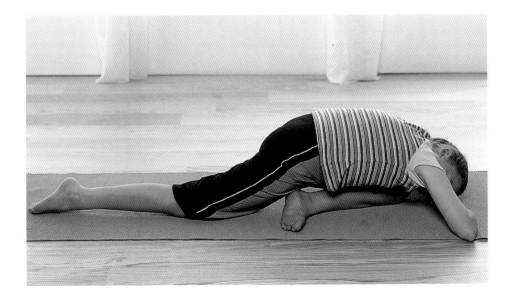

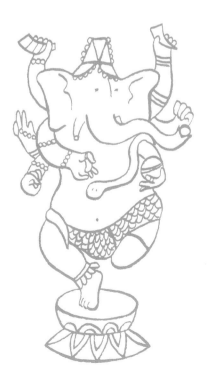

Locust

Shalabhasana

A locust is a tropical grasshopper, with long, strong legs with special springy knees that launch its body into flight. It can jump the equivalent of you jumping over your house! This is a very strong back bend and it may prove too difficult for younger children to hold both legs off the floor. With regular practice it will get easier, but begin by lifting one leg at a time. If you find it too uncomfortable lying on your arms, rest your arms by your sides and rest your forehead on the floor. You can lift your legs in this position too.

benefits

Locust is a challenging pose that strengthens the back muscles. Like other back bends it will also boost your natural energy.

when to do the pose

Practise Locust after you have got the hang of Cobra pose – this will make it easier for you. Follow Locust with a relaxing forward bend such as Child's pose or Sandwich.

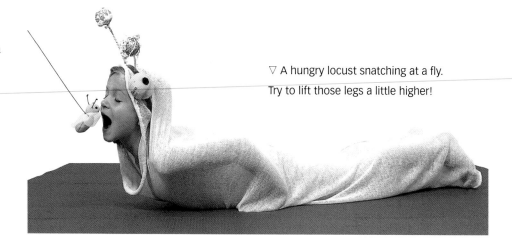

▽ A hungry locust snatching at a fly.
Try to lift those legs a little higher!

a summary of the movements

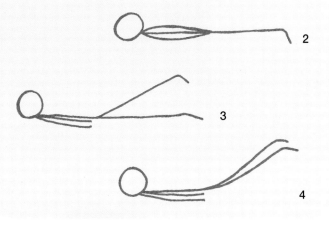

1

2

3

4

1 Lie on your side in a straight line with your arms extended in front of you. Wrap your fingers round the thumb of each hand to make a fist. Bring both of your fists side by side.

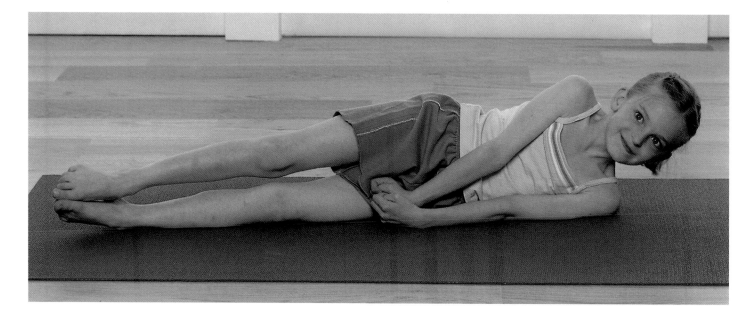

a summary of the movements

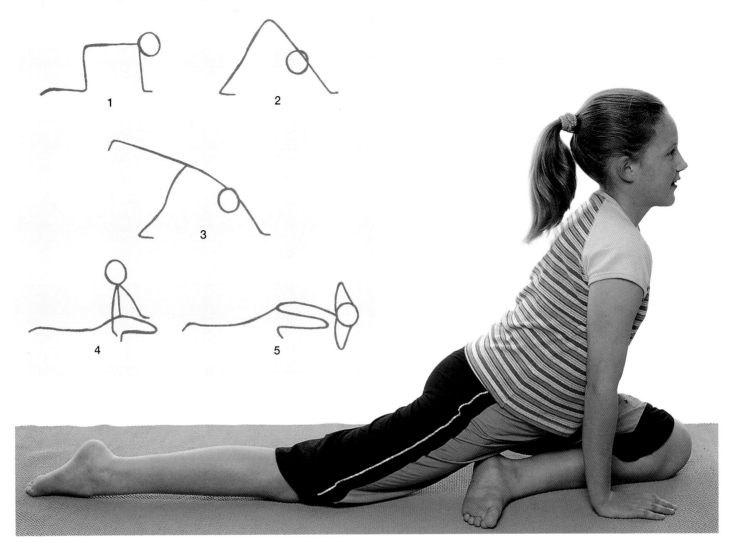

1   2   3   4   5

4 △ Place the knee on the floor and bring the heel to the right. Sit to the outside of your left knee. Let the back of your left thigh release on to the floor. Stretch out your right leg and prop yourself up with your hands.

5 ▽ Breathe steadily and, as you exhale, lean your chest forwards over your knee. Make a pillow with your hands and relax. Close your eyes for a few minutes. Release and rest in Child's pose, then change sides.

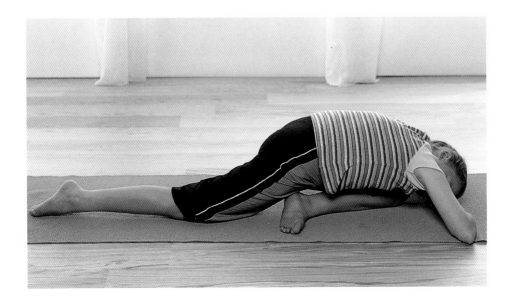

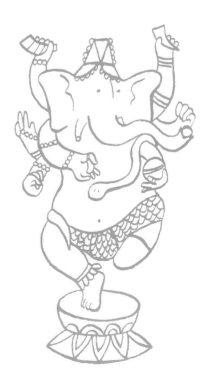

Tortoise

Koormasana

This gentle seated pose will help you to feel the quiet and calmness of a tortoise who knows he is protected by his strong shell. A famous Indian fable called the Bhagavad Gita states that if you can stay safe and calm inside your body, without reacting to danger or difficulty, then, like the tortoise safely inside his protective shell, you will become mighty and wise. This is a useful piece of advice!

benefits

Tortoise pose will make you feel calm and secure because you will imagine yourself protected by a strong shell. This pose will also provide your back and legs with a long stretch.

when to do the pose

Practise Tortoise when you want to feel safe and quiet. It will also help to release your back after a bending pose.

1 Sit on the floor, legs wide apart and bent at the knees. The soles of your feet should be flat on the floor. Your hands can be held in prayer position, or Namaste. Breathe steadily.

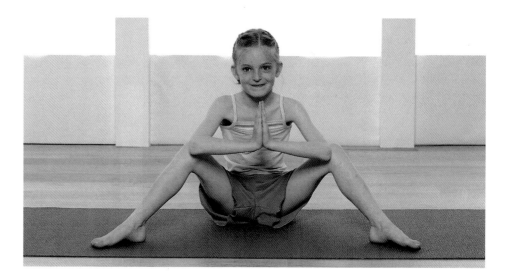

2 As you breathe in, reach up with your right arm, keeping your fingers stretched. Breathe out and feed your right arm underneath your right knee. Hold it there.

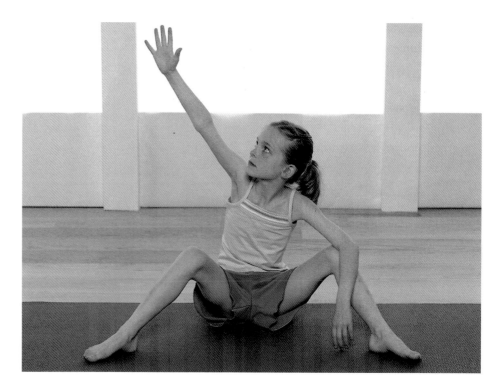

a summary of the movements

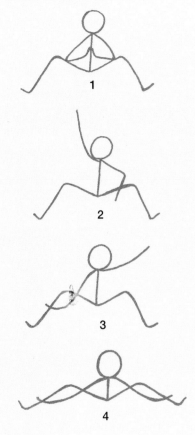

1

2

3

4

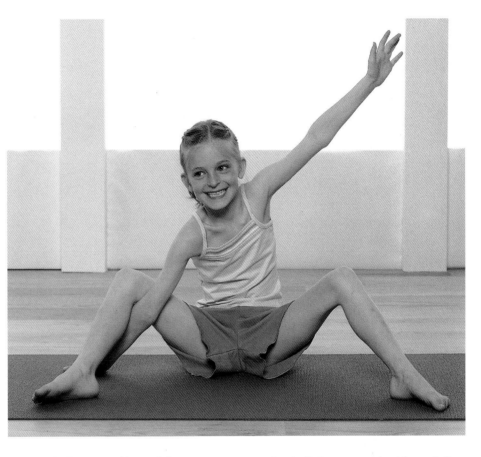

3 Now do the same with your left arm, reaching up and feeding it under your left knee. Breathe steadily.

4 Gradually lower your chest towards the floor as you walk your fingers and hands in the opposite direction to your feet. With practice you may be able to place your chin and chest on the floor in front of you, and straighten your legs on the floor. Slowly release yourself from the position and relax. Have a friend or parent close by to help you unravel yourself from the position.

Locust

Shalabhasana

A locust is a tropical grasshopper, with long, strong legs with special springy knees that launch its body into flight. It can jump the equivalent of you jumping over your house! This is a very strong back bend and it may prove too difficult for younger children to hold both legs off the floor. With regular practice it will get easier, but begin by lifting one leg at a time. If you find it too uncomfortable lying on your arms, rest your arms by your sides and rest your forehead on the floor. You can lift your legs in this position too.

benefits

Locust is a challenging pose that strengthens the back muscles. Like other back bends it will also boost your natural energy.

when to do the pose

Practise Locust after you have got the hang of Cobra pose – this will make it easier for you. Follow Locust with a relaxing forward bend such as Child's pose or Sandwich.

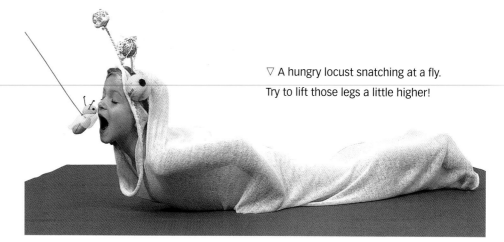

▽ A hungry locust snatching at a fly. Try to lift those legs a little higher!

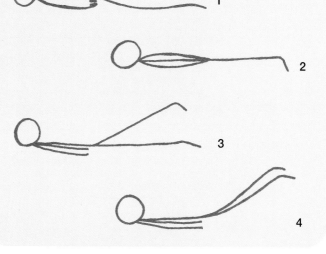

a summary of the movements

1

2

3

4

1 Lie on your side in a straight line with your arms extended in front of you. Wrap your fingers round the thumb of each hand to make a fist. Bring both of your fists side by side.

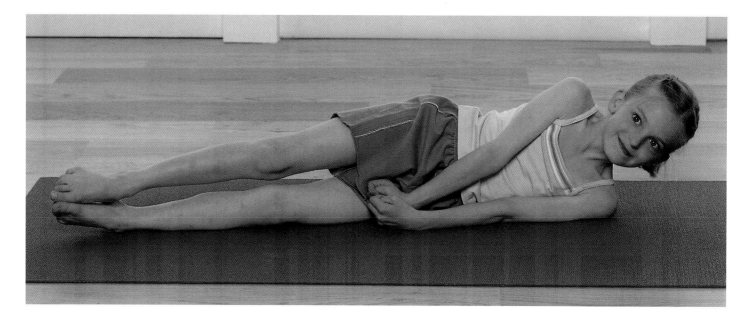

2 Roll gently on to your front so that you are lying on your arms. Wriggle them down as far as you can towards your feet. Let your chin rest on the floor, close your eyes and breathe steadily and deeply to prepare yourself.

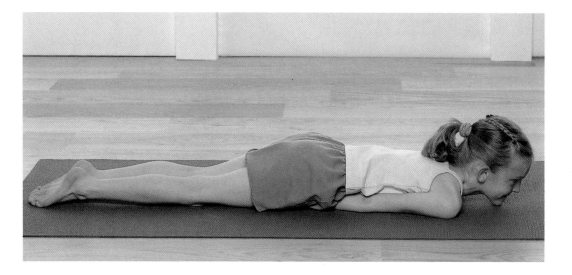

3 Breathe in and lift your right leg off the floor. Push your fists into the ground to help lever the leg upwards. Lower the right leg and, on another breath in, repeat with the left leg. Breathe and hold. Lower the left leg and give yourself a rest.

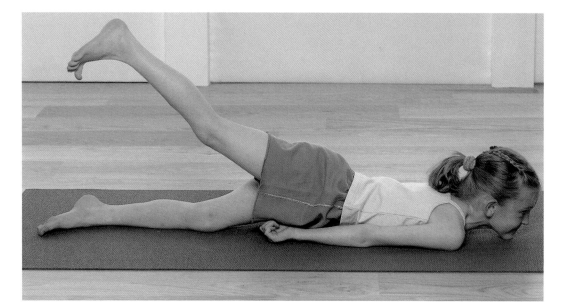

4 When you are ready, take a big breath in and try to lift both legs off the ground. Hold for as long as you can. Gently lower your legs, and come into Child's pose on your knees to relax your back. Well done!

Dragonfly

Sarvangasana

This is a wonderful variation of the classic Shoulder Stand pose. It is known as the queen of yoga postures because of its many physical and holistic qualities. It may look quite hard but when you get into it and have practised a few times you will find that it isn't all that difficult. Resting your knee on your forehead will help you to keep your balance.

benefits of the pose
The Dragonfly pose helps to develop patience and emotional stability. It gives the heart a temporary rest from the effects of gravity, and it feels really wonderful if your legs are heavy and tired. The increased blood flow to your face helps to refresh your brain, and you will find it gives you a big burst of energy.

when to do the pose
Dragonfly is just the thing to do when you come home from a tiring day at school and you feel physically and mentally exhausted and a little bit sluggish. It is good to practise Dragonfly before a dream time sequence, and it can help you to feel emotionally calm and quiet before you go to bed at night.

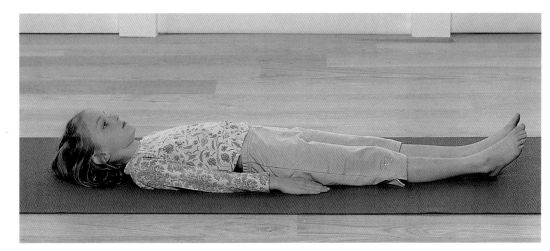

1 Lie flat on your back in Dead Man's pose, with your arms by your sides. Breathe steadily.

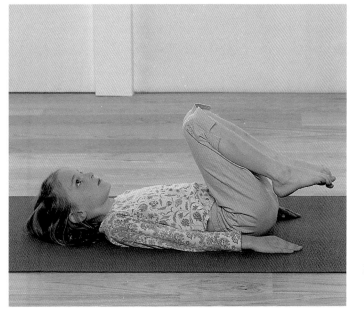

2 Slowly bring your knees in towards your chest, keeping your arms in position at your sides. Continue to breathe steadily.

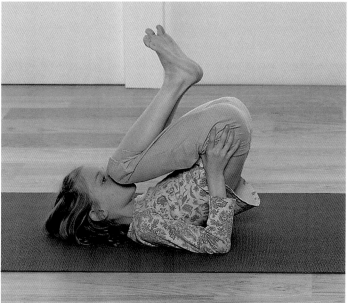

3 Then slowly draw your knees in towards your forehead by pushing your hips and lower back towards you. Use your hands to guide you, then support your back with your flat palms.

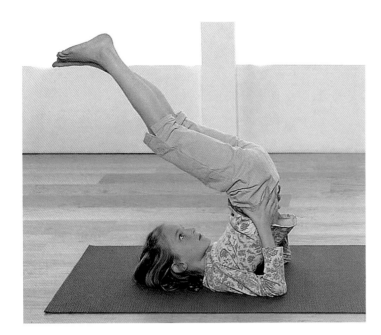

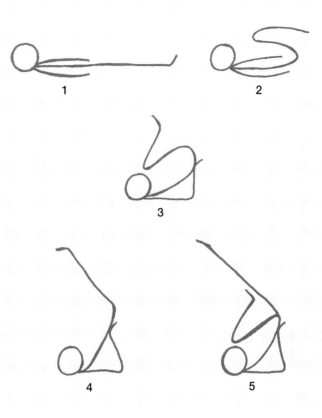

4 Still supporting your lower back, extend your legs upwards so that your toes are directly above you. Hold here and breathe while you get your balance and get used to being upside down.

5 Bend your right knee and rest it in the middle of your forehead. Let the front of your left leg rest on the sole of the right foot. Close your eyes and rest in the pose, keeping your breathing quiet and steady. Change legs when you are ready. Then bring both knees in towards your chest and roll back down on to the floor. Extend your legs and rest on your back.

Cow

Gomukasana

In India the cow is considered a sacred animal, and is allowed to wander the roads on its own. In this seated pose, your body is supposed to resemble the face of this beloved creature. Your stacked knees form the lips of its face and your raised elbow is one of its ears. Practise the pose in stages, if you like. Begin by sitting with just your legs crossed until you feel comfortable, then practise kneeling with your arms in position. When you are happy to sit like this you can move on to the full Cow position.

benefits

Cow pose will release tight muscles in the area around your hips and bottom. It opens up the chest, which will improve your posture, and can also help to release and realign tight or rounded shoulders.

when to do the pose

This is a great pose to do when your hips and shoulders feel stiff from tiredness, too much sitting or too much exercise. It is a good pose to do when you want to challenge yourself. Because you end up looking like a cow's face, it will also make you laugh.

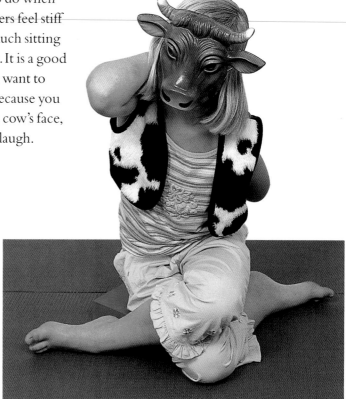

▷ Don't tie yourself in knots over Cow pose. Take it easy and build up the positions in stages.

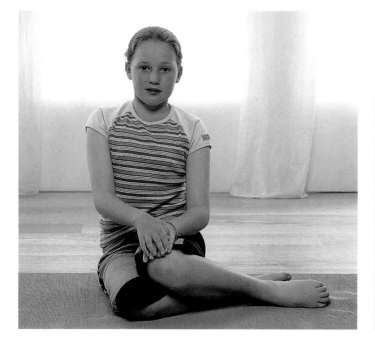

1 Sit down on the floor with your legs to one side and folded to the left of you. Hold one hand over the other and rest them on your top knee. Steady your breathing.

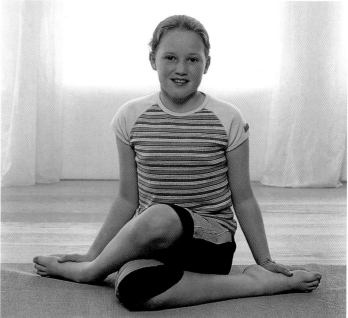

2 Lift up your left leg and cross it over your right knee, so that your knees are now on top of each other. Wriggle your bottom a little so that it is sitting flat on the floor.

▽ You can give yourself an additional stretch by bending your body forwards over your knees. Breathe deeply and hold for a moment.

a summary of the movements

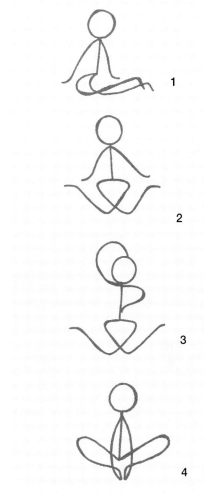

1

2

3

4

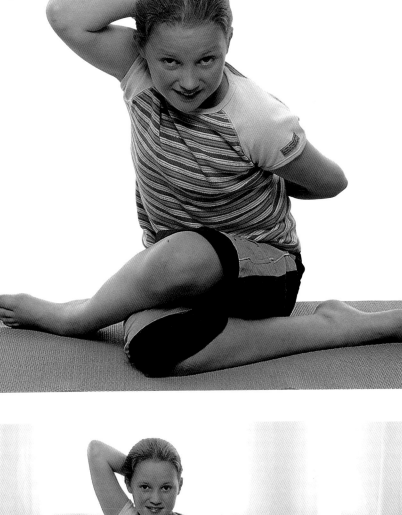

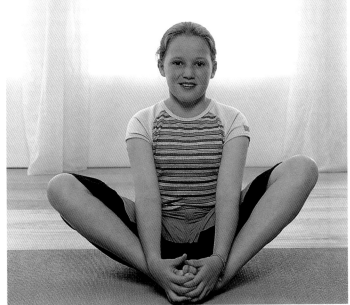

3 Reach up with your right arm and rest your fingers at the base of your neck. Place your left arm behind your back and wriggle it up to meet your other hand. Try to interlink your fingers without rounding your back. Catch hold of your T-shirt if you can't reach. Breathe deeply.

4 Slowly unravel your legs and arms and come into Butterfly pose to relax the muscles. Have a short rest, and change sides whenever you are ready.

Camel

Ushtrasana

This pose is performed on the knees and involves arching carefully backwards so that you make the rounded hump of the camel with your upper body. The arch of the back is particularly important for Camel, so practise getting this part right.

benefits

Camel pose opens up the chest and the heart, and this helps to correct poor or lazy posture. It can help all children to stand tall and feel proud of who they are. Camel encourages good use of the lungs and aids digestion.

when to do the pose

Camel pose is good when you have been working hard, bent over your desk all day at school. It is also good when you want to wake up your back muscles, and when your energy levels are low and need a boost.

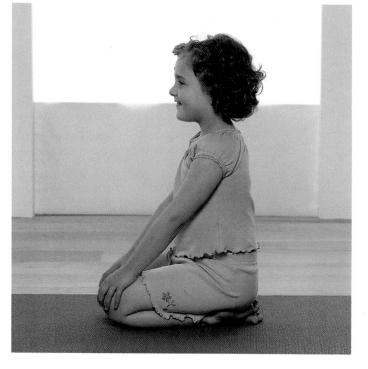

1 Kneel on the floor with your knees hip-width apart. Breathe steadily and deeply for a few minutes.

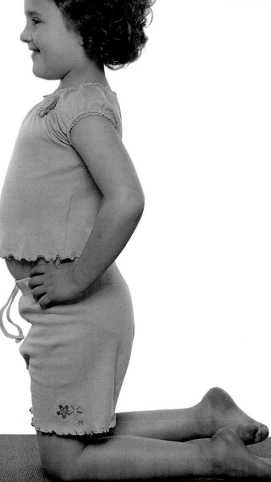

2 Then sit up and look straight ahead of you, bringing your hands on to your hips.

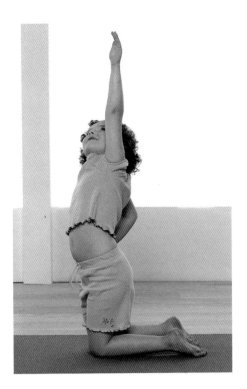

3 Tuck under your toes so that your heels lift up off the floor, then breathe in and lift your left arm upwards. Look up at your hand.

a summary of the movements

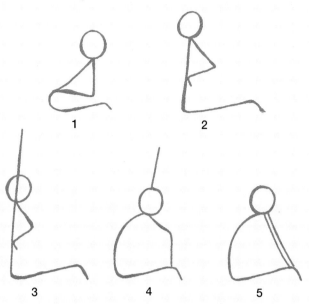

1   2

3   4   5

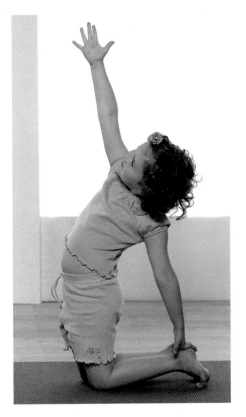

4 ◁ Circle your left arm round and rest your fingertips on your left heel. Keep pushing your heart and chest forwards. Lift your right arm in the same way.

5 ▷ Circle your right arm round behind you and bring your fingertips on to your right heel. Breathe in and out steadily, pushing your chest proudly forwards to make the camel's hump.

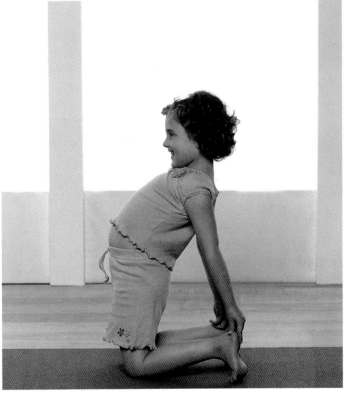

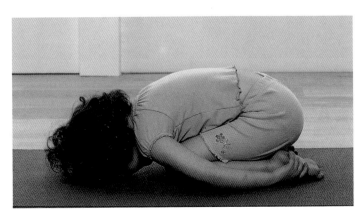

6 Release and lean forwards in Child's pose to rest your back. Sit down on your heels and rest your forehead on the floor in front of you, with your arms by your sides.

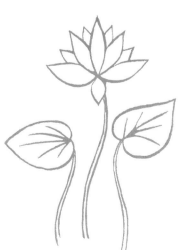

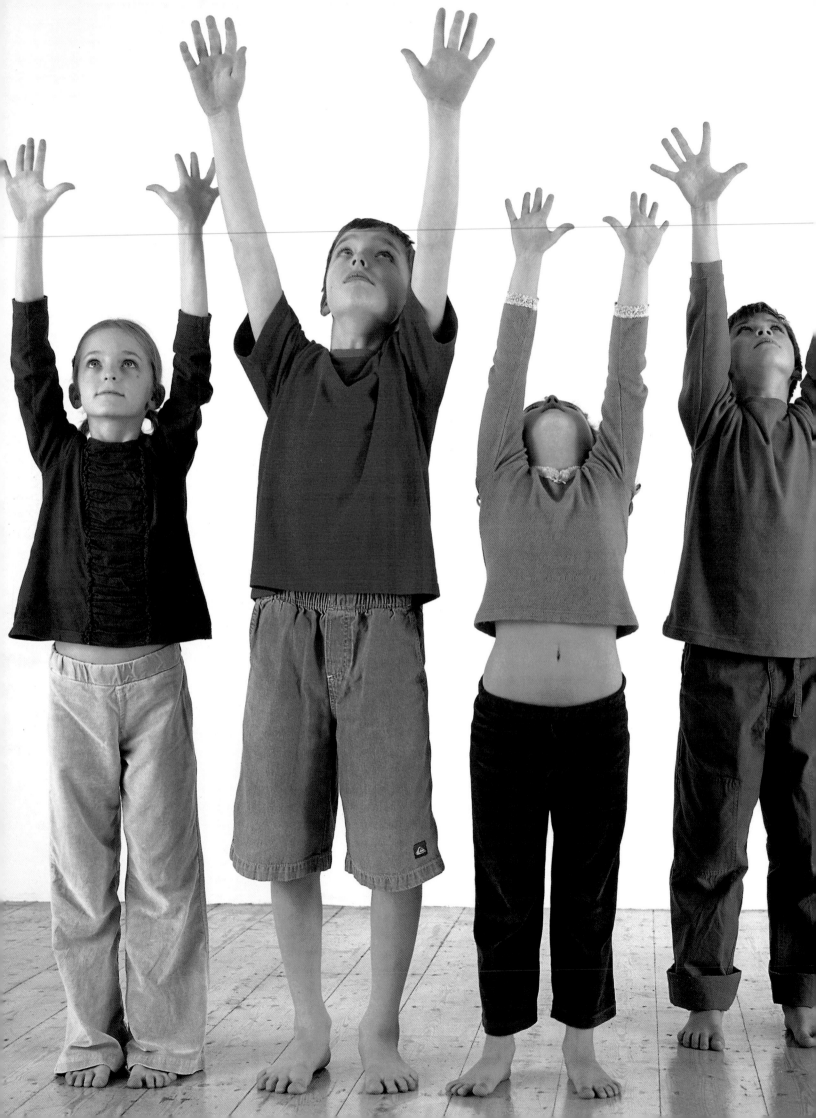

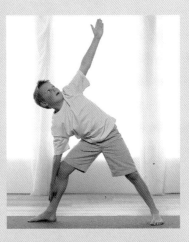

putting
it all
together

Here we show you how to build the

stand-alone poses you have learnt into

flowing themed sequences, to help you

discover new and more challenging poses.

There are three of these for you to try, as

well as a yoga play, and all are lovely ways

of showcasing your new skills to friends

and family. As your confidence grows,

try making up and naming your own

poses. Simply remember to practise them

slowly and mindfully, breathing deeply

and steadily at all times.

Your postures: make them up

Just as the first yogis created postures from studying the world around them, you too can get creative and make up some of your own. Inventing postures is a wonderful way to stimulate your imagination. It will also help to keep you interested by showing you how much you can adapt yoga to suit your mood.

Think about creatures or objects that inspire you. It could be magical creatures from story books, such as fairies and unicorns, gremlins and ghosts, or favourite animals, birds or insects seen in the garden, on holiday or studied at school. Think about how these animals move, sleep and hunt. Are they big or small, fast or slow, gentle or dangerous?

In addition to the animal kingdom, use the modern world as a source of inspiration. Try the Aeroplane pose below, or think about other modes of transport and how you could imitate

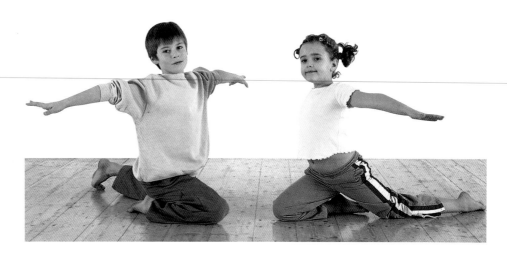

them. How would you translate a silent, slow-moving submarine into a yoga pose? What about a sailing boat?

Remember to do the poses slowly and to keep breathing while you do them. If you are feeling really creative, think about what type of pose should come after the one you have made up. These are the counter poses that help your body erase the last posture and move it in the opposite way, allowing it to rebalance itself.

△ **Seagulls** Kneel on one knee with one leg outstretched and your arms spread to your sides. Imagine warm sea air rising up under your wings, helping you to glide in the air.

▽ **Aeroplanes** This is a strong pose and is very good for your legs. Stand up tall with your hands in prayer position. Breathe in and, as you breathe out, lunge one leg forwards. Spread your arms (or wings) out to the sides and drop your chest towards your front knee. Enjoy the flight, then change legs.

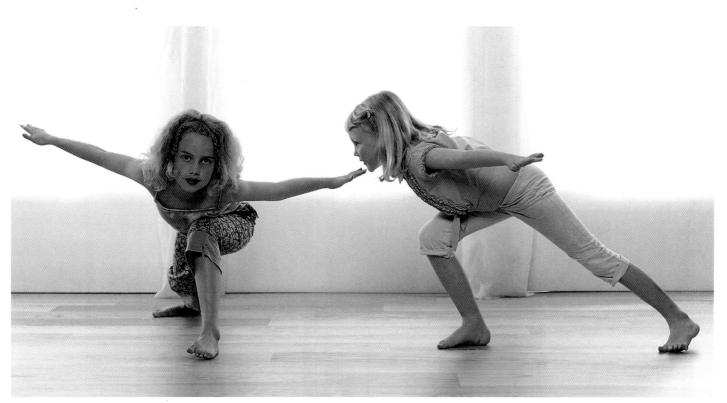

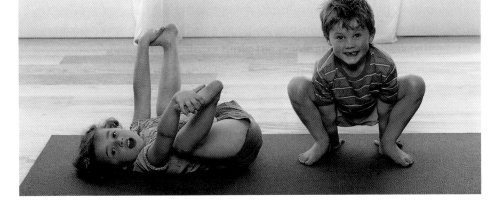

◁ **Beetle and sparrow** The upturned beetle, here on the left, must roll out of the way of the hungry chirping sparrow.

▽ **Rag dolls** Stand up straight with your feet hip-width apart. Hang your head and let your body and arms fall gently forwards like a drooping flower or a floppy rag doll as it is lifted from the toy box.

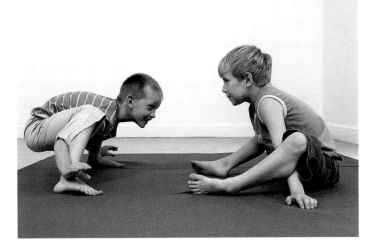

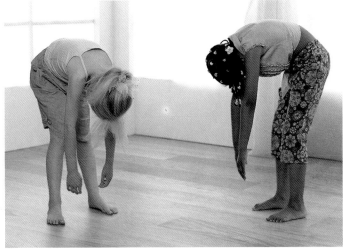

△ **Animal antics** See if you can squat down low like a spider. Which one of you will be the first to collapse?

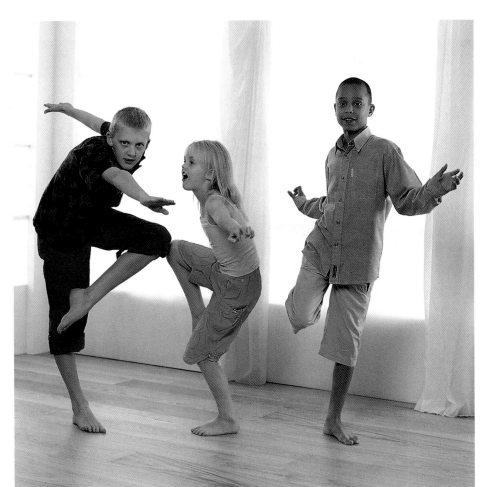

▷ **Cactus plants** Stand up straight and lift one knee so that you are balancing on one leg. Angle your arms and legs to make the eerie shapes of prickly cactus plants…but don't touch or it could hurt!

▷

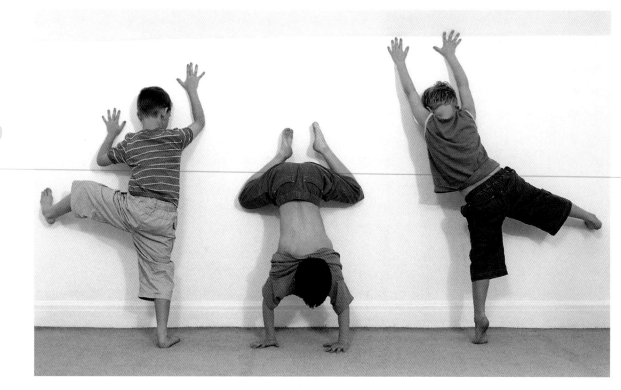

◁ **Geckos** Use your body to imitate the nimble movements of a gecko – which is a type of lizard – as he clings to a wall. Stretch out your arms and legs, spread your fingers and toes and hang on.

Dragon

This is a pose for two people. As it involves one person carrying the other on their back, it helps if the supporter is an adult. Roaring and fire-breathing are optional!

1 The supporter sits on her knees with her forehead on the floor and both her arms stretched out in front. The child lies across her back, and stretches out his arms and legs. It may take a few attempts for you both to find your balance and hold the position.

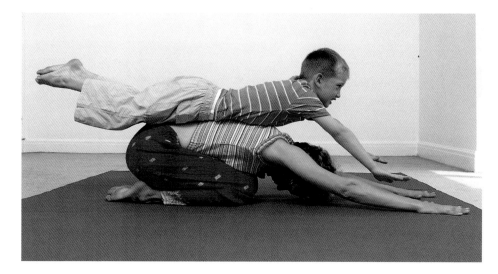

2 The child on top takes hold of his partner's arms and holds on tight. He tucks his toes under and lifts his back. The dragon then stretches out his legs and gets a wonderful ride, while the supporter strengthens her arms, wrists and legs. Hold still, or lower and lift as many times as you can while the dragon roars. Relax.

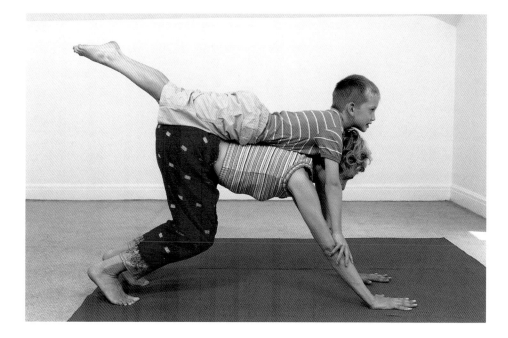

Elephant walk

The more of you the merrier for this one as you imitate the lumbering, trunk-swinging swagger of a herd of elephants.

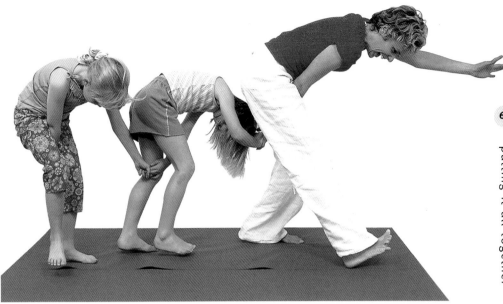

1 Stand in line, one behind the other. All of you now reach forwards. Put one arm between your legs to make a tail and grasp the hand of the elephant behind you. Hold out your other arm in front of you to make a trunk and grasp the hand of the elephant in front.

2 Make sure you are all connected in this way, then amble slowly forwards, with your feet stomping and trunks trumpeting.

3 Continue stomping and trumpeting your way round and round the room or the garden. Release your hands and and relax, straightening up your back and stretching your arms up above your head.

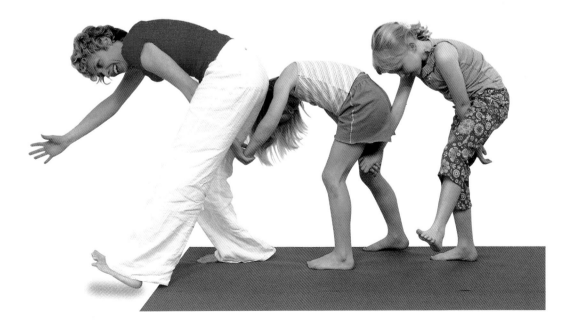

I am strong

Developing stamina and strength helps us to feel the amazing power of our physical body. We have all felt the sense of elation that follows physical activity. These poses are empowering, and are designed to build confidence.

give it some muscle!

It is through our musculoskeletal system that we experience the physical potential of our bodies. It also gives us the sense of how strong we judge ourselves to be. This system of muscles and bones works as a team to give us an extraordinary range of movement and a sense of inner power.

Strong yoga poses – particularly those that support our body weight on either our feet or hands – keep muscles and bones in peak condition. Bones renew themselves and continue to grow only in response to such weight-bearing activity. Muscles like to be stretched gently and smoothly and supplied with as much oxygen as possible. Coming into these poses slowly, and breathing deeply and steadily as you hold them, allows the the body to move in a natural way. This gives your muscles a lovely slow, non-violent stretch, and builds solidity and strength in your bones.

emotional strength

Emotional strength is important, too. It means that we can stand on our own two feet and deal with the knocks of life and still come up smiling. The drive to succeed and persevere is rooted in a natural instinct for survival deep inside us. These strong poses can help children to access this instinct and deepen their inner conviction and drive.

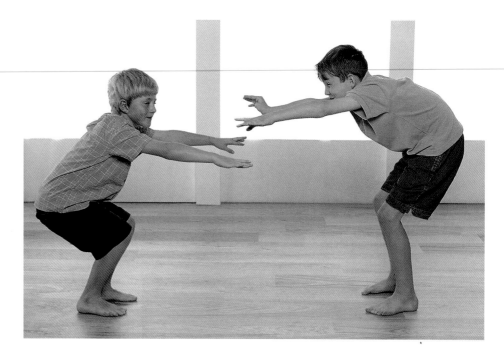

△ **Chair or fierce pose** Stand with your legs together, feet firm. Exhale and bend your knees as if you were sitting on an invisible chair, arms down by your side. Breathe in and lift your arms out in front of you at shoulder height. Hold the position and breathe. To release, roll your body forwards into the Rag Doll pose.

Woodchopper

This pose is fun and will quickly fill you with energy. You can also do it when you are in need of some inspiration. Repeat three or four times until you feel full of energy.

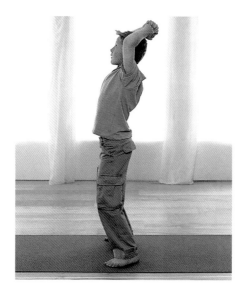

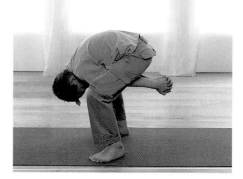

1 Stand with feet hip-width apart, and your knees gently bent. Make a strong fist with both of your hands together, and as you breathe in, lift the fist over your head.

2 Swing the axe through your legs, keeping your knees bent, and exhale through your mouth with a loud "Haaa!". Breathe in and lift your hands over your head again. Repeat.

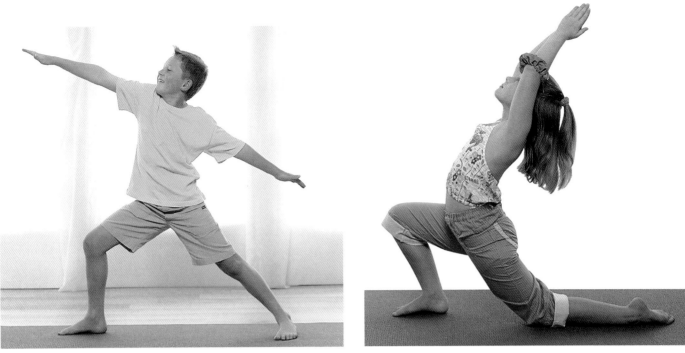

△ **Warrior** Step your feet wide apart and bend your front knee over your ankle, with the front foot facing forwards and the back foot turned away by 30°. Breathe in and lift both arms to the sides. Breathe out and bend your front knee a little more. Look at your front hand. Feel the strength growing in your legs. Release and change sides.

▷ **Triangle** Position your feet in the same way as for Warrior and stand sideways, this time with both legs straight. Lift your arms to the side as you breathe in and, as you breathe out, reach as far over your front foot as you can. Inhale, then drop your hand down to touch your lower leg as you breathe out. Look up at your other hand and hold for a few deep breaths. Release and change sides. It may be easier for little children to think of this pose as a teapot.

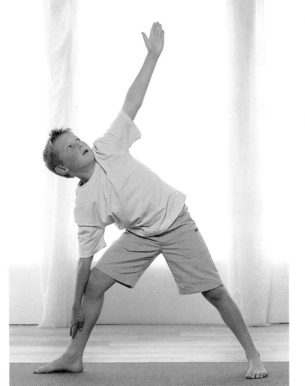

△ **Crescent moon** Kneel on the floor with your bottom off your heels and your back straight. Step your right foot forwards at a right angle to your left leg. Inhale and, as you exhale, push your right knee upright over your right foot. Inhale again and lift your arms over your head into prayer position. As you breathe out, arch your back to make a lovely curved C-shape from your fingers to your toes. Push your back foot into the floor to keep you steady, and hold. Slowly release and change sides. Rest for a few minutes in Child's pose to rebalance your body, bending forwards over your knees.

▽ **Wheel** Lie on your back with your knees bent and your feet hip-width apart. Raise your arms behind your head, bend them and place your palms flat on the floor with your fingertips tucking in below your shoulders. Take a deep breath and exhale with an "Aahh!" sound as you push into your hands and lift your bottom off the floor. Take a few deep breaths. Lower your back to the floor. Relax and hug your knees.

Jungle walk

Setting your yoga session in an imaginary location such as the jungle gives you plenty of scope for having fun, and lets the children delight at becoming the wild creatures and characters they may find there.

First the children must prepare for their jungle journey, shrugging and rolling their shoulders as if to put on imaginary rucksacks, and flexing and pointing their toes to put on their big, strong jungle boots.

Walk through the trees, scanning the horizon for wild animals. Walk on tiptoe to look over the tall grass, and stomp through muddy swamps. Introduce an array of animals and spend some time imitating each one.

1 Lunge forwards as you set off and look all around you. Who knows what creatures may be hiding in the trees!

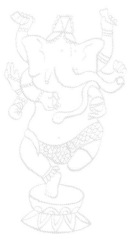

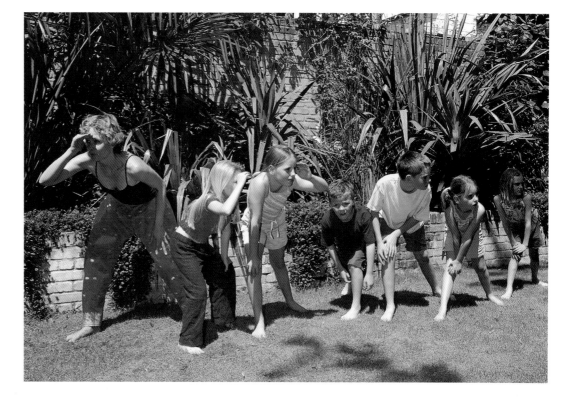

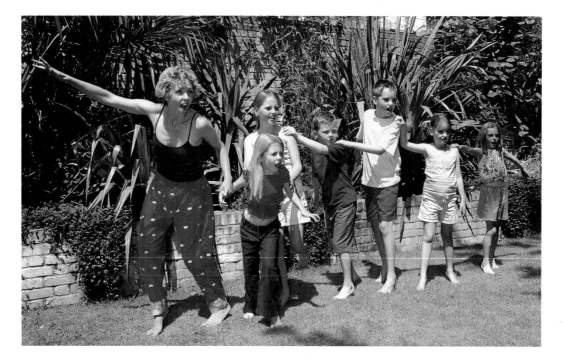

2 Tiptoe quietly through the tall grass. Keep a hand on the shoulder of the person in front of you to make sure no one gets left behind.

3 ▽ Look over there, there's an elephant! See his long trunk! Where is the rest of his herd?

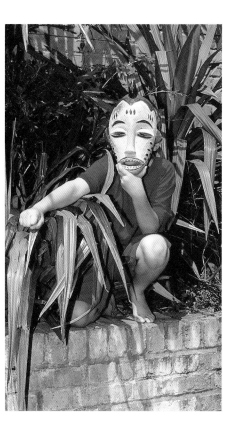

4 ▷ Now strike a pose as a fierce jungle warrior to make yourself feel more brave.

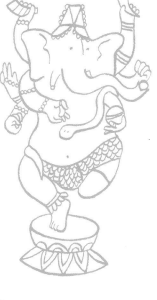

5 Watch out everyone! Over there in the trees are a couple of lions. Let's hope they aren't hungry!

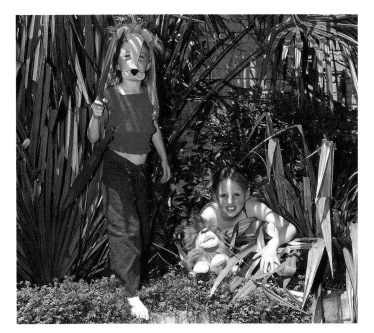

6 Once the group is safely back at the camp you can make a fire to warn away the wild animals. All sit in a circle on the floor and lie on your backs. Raise your legs and bring your feet together to make the flames of a fire in Candle pose.

Dolphin dive

The ocean fills children with wonder and awe, and marine life and seaside activities can be used to explore a host of exciting new yoga poses.

From the big fish that live in the sea, such as dolphins, whales and sharks, to magical, mythical mermaids and the curious creatures that hide in rock pools, there are plenty of sea-life characters to choose from. Create your own sea-life poses. You could be a catfish, dogfish, seal or sea lion – The possibilities are endless.

high tide, low tide

Spend time doing strong, active poses until you feel you have had enough and are ready to quieten the pace. Dressing up will add to the fun.

As your energy levels begin to drop, introduce poses that will allow you to relax. Play soothing music inspired by the sounds of the sea, and curl up in Child's pose: sitting on your heels and resting your head on the floor in front of you, with your arms lying relaxed by your sides. Tell yourself that you are a small, smooth pebble that has been tossed by the sea waves and washed up on the beach. Then, after a few minutes' rest, wake yourself gently, as if you were a cautious hermit crab peering out of his shell…

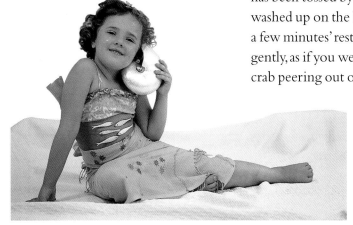

◁ **Mermaid** Think of yourself as a little mermaid, living on the ocean floor with seashells and pearls for your toys.

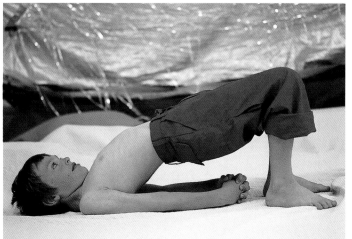

△ **Seahorse** Sit on your knees with your bottom off the floor. Stretch upwards so that your back is straight, and lift your arms and hands to make the elegant long neck of a seahorse. Hold the position and breathe deeply for a few breaths. Relax.

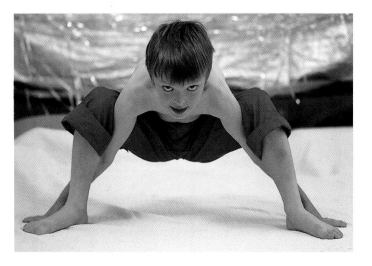

△ **Crab** Squat down with your legs wide apart and place your hands on the floor, one behind each leg. Lift your head and beady eyes and look around you. Now scuttle from side to side. See how high you can lift one arm or leg, like a defiant claw!

△ **Blue whale** Lie on your back with your legs bent and your feet flat on the floor. Think of your tummy as the blue whale's back and your navel as its blowhole. Breathe in and, as you breathe out, lift up your bottom high off the floor. Try lifting one leg to flip your mighty tail.

▷ **Dolphin** Get down on the floor on your hands and knees. Place your elbows on the floor under your shoulders and interlace your fingers to make a fist. Curl your toes under and push your bottom up into the air. Keep breathing gently. To swim, dip your chin over the fist as you breathe in, then lift it back again as you breathe out. Keep going until you have had enough, then rest.

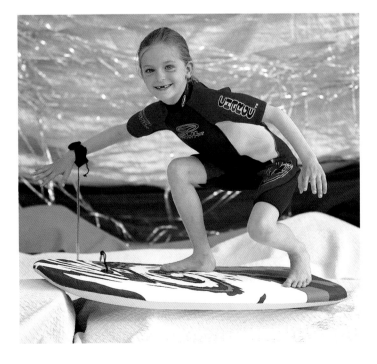

◁ Stand with your feet together and your hands by your sides to be a surfer. Breathe in and, as you breathe out, jump your feet so that they are hip-width apart and bend your knees into a semi-squatting position. Lift your arms for balance and visualize yourself riding the crest of a wave. Change sides after a few long breaths.

▷ Dolphins are flexible and strong, and they have a lot of fun dipping and diving through the ocean waves.

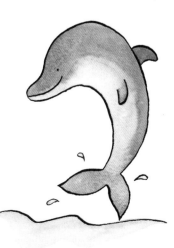

Moon meandering

The moon is a magical setting that appeals hugely to the imagination of children. It is the perfect setting to explore a galaxy of new yoga poses.

You can add to the drama of the moon location by doing these poses in a darkened room with soft lighting, and by adding silver accessories to whatever you are wearing. Try to really imagine what it would be like to be a spaceman, stepping over the craters of the moon for the first time. Or what it would be like to be a sparkling star twinkling down on children and creatures as they sleep.

The Moon

The squalling cat and the squeaking mouse
The howling dog by the door of the house
The bat that lies in bed at noon
All love to be out by the light of the moon

Robert Louis Stevenson

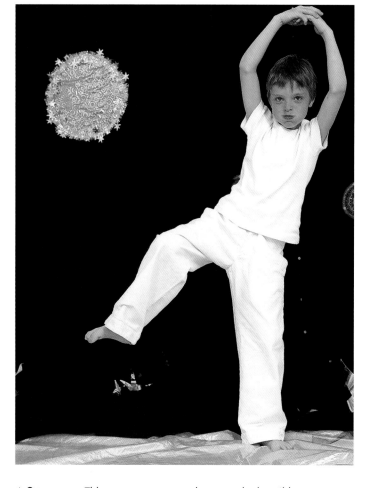

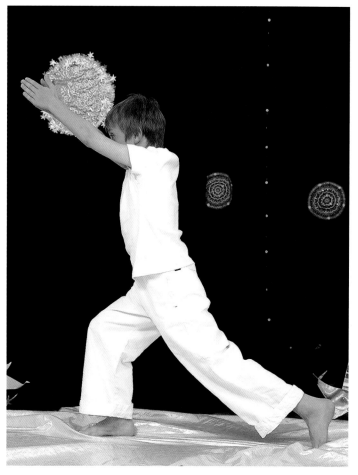

△ **Spaceman** This pose encourages deep, regular breathing as you make the helmet of your space suit with your arms above your head. Imagine what your breath would sound like inside a big bubble helmet. Lift one leg and balance while you breathe, then change sides.

△ **Moon walking** Do Spaceman's pose and then with your heavy feet in big silver space boots, begin to take big, lunging steps as if you were walking over the surface of the moon. Try to synchronize your footsteps with your breath.

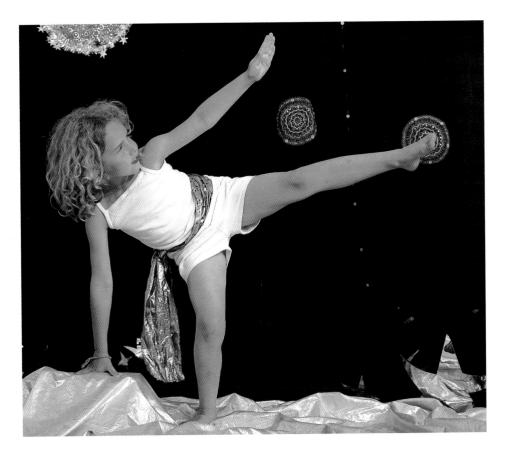

◁ **Half moon** Stand side-on to a chair or low ledge, about 0.5m (2ft) away from you. Drop your right arm down to the support. In time you may not need this and will be able to drop your hand straight to the floor. Lift your left leg up and balance on one leg and arm. Now lift your left arm up. Look up towards it if you can, breathing steadily. Release and change sides.

▽ **Twinkling star** Make the points of a star with your legs and arms outstretched. Feel as tall and wide as you can. Imagine light spreading outwards from your tummy button and into your fingers and toes.

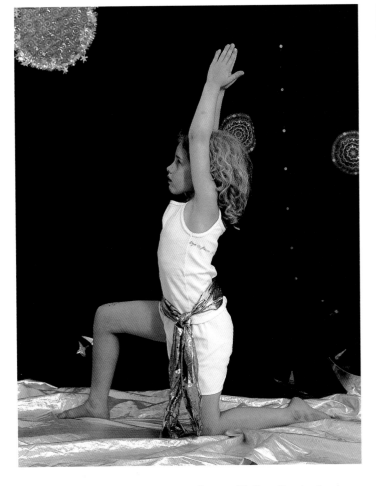

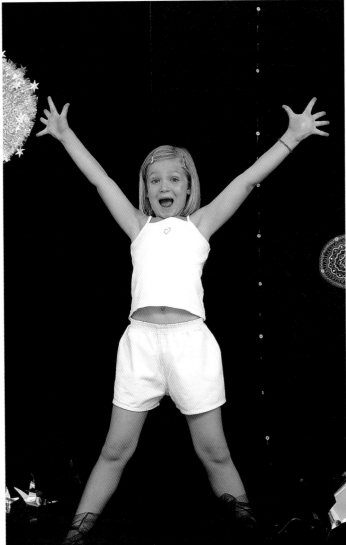

△ **Space rocket** Kneel down on one knee, with the other leg bent in front of you. Breathe in and lift your arms up over your head. Press your palms together to make the top of your rocket, and stretch as tall as you can, as if you are about to be launched into space.

A yoga play

All that is required for a yoga play is a simple story or sequence of events that can be acted out using yoga poses. Think about your favourite stories, nursery rhymes or poems as a starting point, particularly those that feature a good selection of interesting animals or characters. Gather a group of your friends together and ask yourselves who or what you would like to be, then try to get into character. Older children, with a more developed imagination, may prefer to invent their own stories and yoga poses, but smaller children relate best to stories and ideas they are familiar with.

When you have rehearsed your play, create a mock stage at home and invite other members of your family and their friends to come and watch.

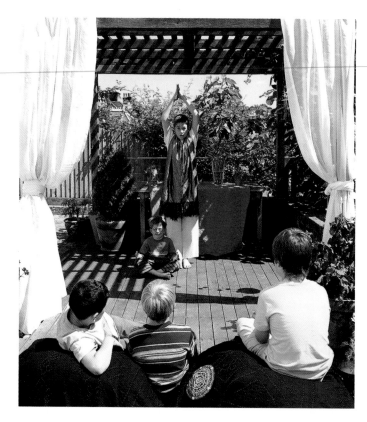

1 Once upon a time there was a wise old wizard and his mischievous, young son, whose name was Little Buddha. They lived deep in the forest in a far away land.

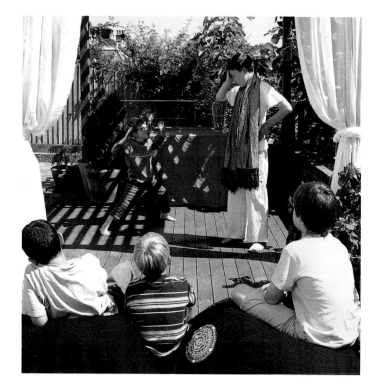

2 Little Buddha was mostly a well-behaved boy, but one day he was bored and he decided to rebel! His poor father scratched his head in despair. Whatever could he do with Little Buddha?

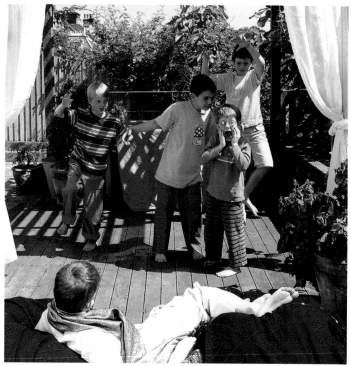

3 But it was too late! Little Buddha ran off and travelled a long, long way, deep into the forest. It was a dark place, full of twisted trees, wicked beasts and strange noises, and he became very scared.

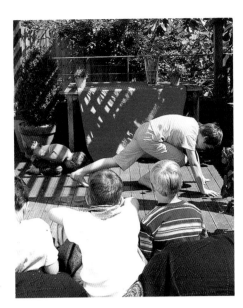

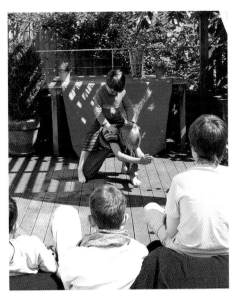

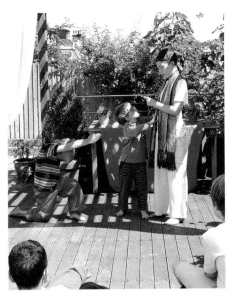

4 Whenever one of the wicked beasts came up to him, Little Buddha dropped to the floor and froze like a smooth, round pebble. He found that this would make the scary beasts go away again.

5 Little Buddha was pleased with his new skills. He had no intention of returning home now that he could protect himself. Then a majestic unicorn appeared. He carried Little Buddha away on his back and told him he was taking him to a beautiful princess.

6 But it was a trick! When they stopped there was no princess. It was his father, who had used his wizard powers to find his son. His father was very cross and told Little Buddha he must return home immediately.

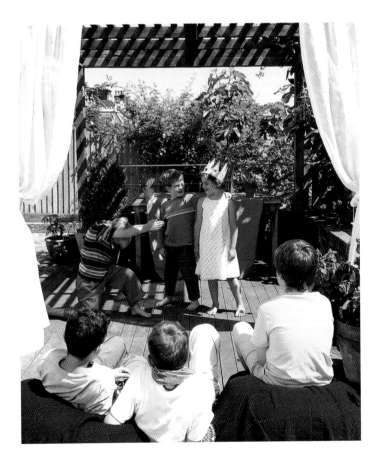

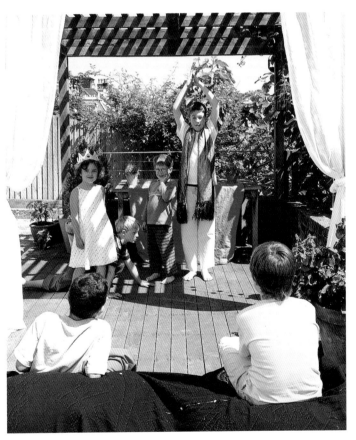

7 Little Buddha was furious and refused. He had fallen in love with the idea of the princess and would return only with her. Suddenly, the unicorn reappeared, carrying the princess. She really did exist!

8 The princess smiled at Little Buddha, and it made him feel sorry for not listening to his father. He had learnt his lesson at last, and so he and the princess and the unicorn returned home with the wizard. And of course they all lived happily ever after!

The End

Yoga games

Yoga postures can be very easily incorporated into many traditional children's games. All that is called for is a little imagination and modification. Using games in this way is a clever way of keeping children's enthusiasm for yoga practice alive. Games are also an ideal activity for when friends come round to play, and in fact, the more children the better.

You may recognize the classic games that have been adapted in this section. Copy Me is a version of Simon Says and the idea for Wise Man Walk has come from Grandmother's Footsteps.

Copy me

Appoint a leader to call out the yoga poses. The group must only perform the posture when the leader says "Copy me!" followed by the name of the pose. Anyone who makes three mistakes is out of the game.

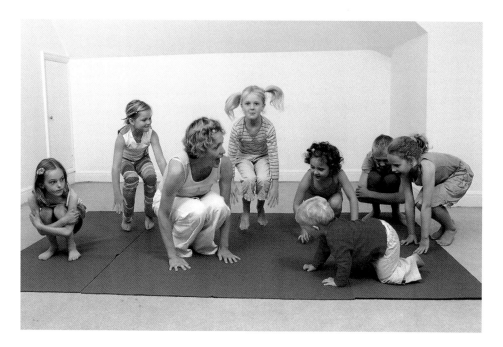

1 Copy me and squat like a rabbit! Everyone squat on the floor and hop up and down.

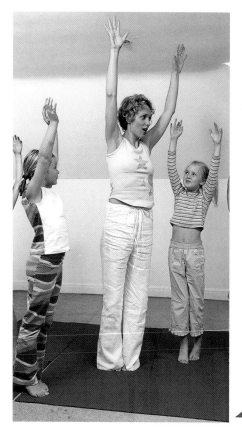

2 ◁ Copy me and be as tall as a mountain! Everyone put your arms in the air and stretch out your fingers to make yourself tall.

3 ▽ Copy me and hoot like an owl! Form "O" shapes with your fingers to make big, wide owl eyes.

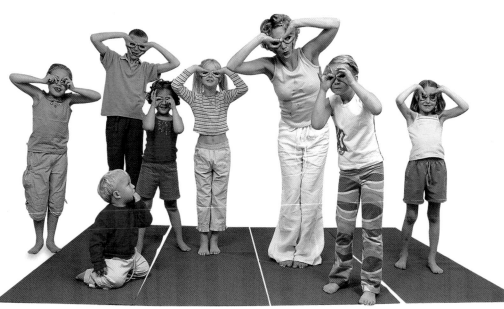

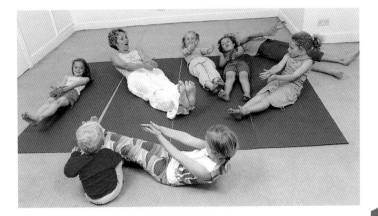

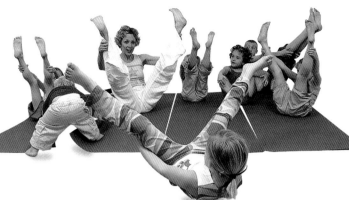

5 ▽ Copy me and be a tall ship! Now all lean back, and hold your legs out wide to make the sails of your ship. Feel the wind in your sails as you try to keep your balance.

4 △ Copy me and be a seal! Everyone sit down on the floor and stretch out your legs, lifting them slightly off the floor to make your tail. Extend your arms in front of you to make your flippers.

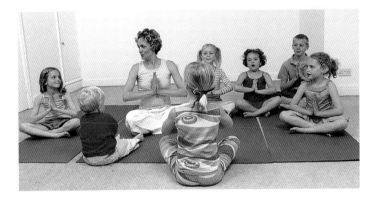

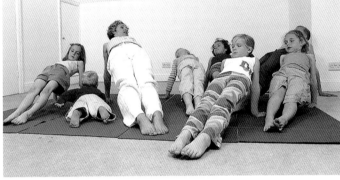

6 △ Copy me and be a Little Buddha! Everyone sit with their legs crossed and their hands in prayer position, with palms flat together. Try to keep those backs straight!

7 △ Copy me and be a slippery slide! Now everyone stretch out your legs and point your toes. Push up with your hands to lift your bottoms off the floor.

8 ◁ Copy me and stand in Mountain pose. Then squat down slowly to the floor. Uh-oh, out you go!

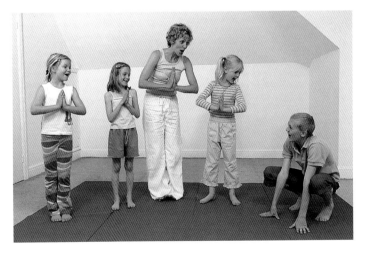

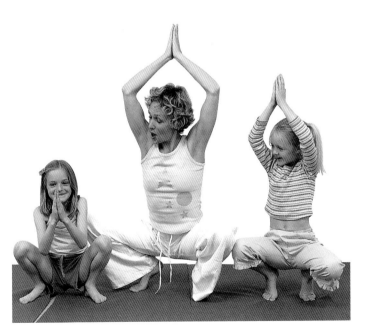

9 ◁ Copy me and be a snake! Lie down on your front with your legs outstretched behind you. Push down into your hands and lift your chest and head strongly upwards.

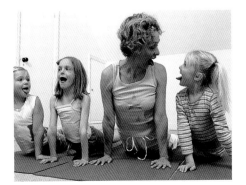

10 △ Copy me and jump up into squatting! Squat down on the balls of your feet and lift your hands up above your head, with your palms together in prayer position. Oh no, you're out!

▷

Snap and snack

This group game involves a cluster of crocodiles lying side by side. Choose an intrepid explorer to step gingerly over the sleepy crocodiles without touching them. If he or she fails, the crocodiles arch up with tails swishing and teeth snapping and the explorer is out. Try this game as seals too, lying on your backs.

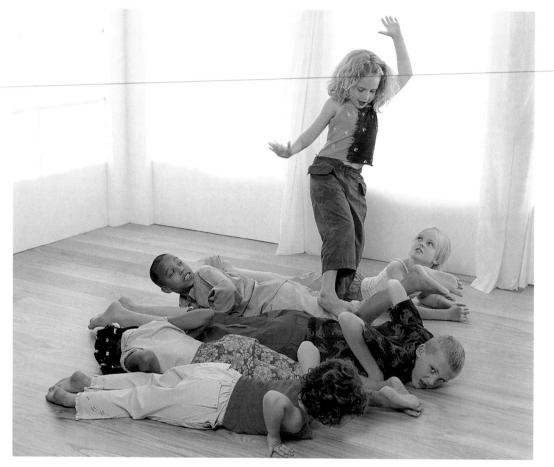

◁ **Crocodiles** Come into Crocodile pose by lying on your front and bringing your legs together to make the heavy tail. Bring your hands underneath your shoulders and place your palms flat on the floor. These are your clawed feet. Look out for that unwanted visitor. SNAP!

▷ **Seals** These lazy snoozing seals will soon let you know if you've woken them up. Watch out for their noisy barking and flapping fins if you touch them.

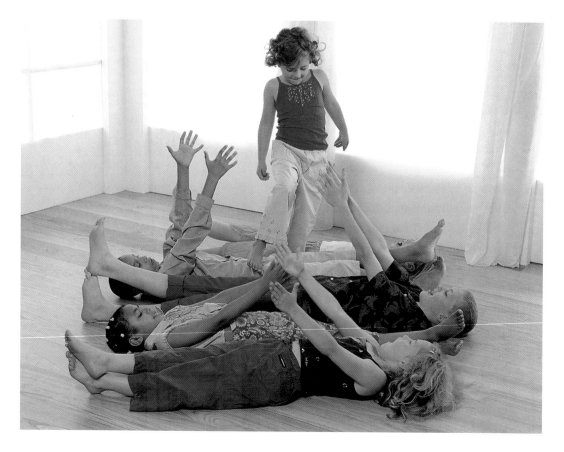

Wise man walk

This involves a group of wise men and a watcher, who stands with his back to the group. The wise men can only move when they are not being watched, and must freeze in a posture when the watcher turns round. If anyone moves when the watcher turns, the whole group goes back to the start.

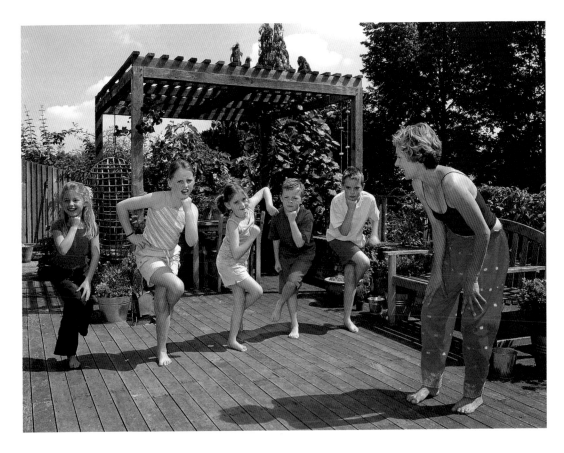

1 Offer a choice of postures before the game starts. When the group is ready, the watcher shouts out, "Everybody become an eagle!" The group of wise men now have to take up the posture. From a standing position, bend your knees and cross one leg over the other. Make a fist and place it under your chin. Support your elbow with the palm of your other hand, and try to balance.

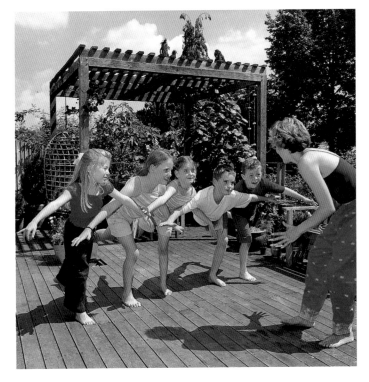

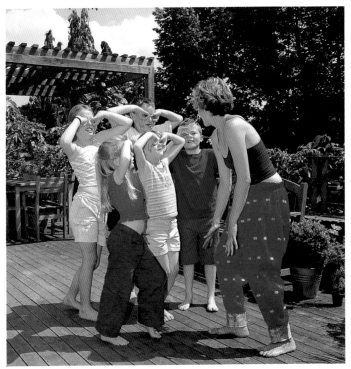

2 When the watcher shouts "Everybody become an aeroplane!", stand up tall and breathe in. As you breathe out, balance on one leg and lift one leg behind you. Spread your arms out to the sides (for the aeroplane's wings) and drop your chest towards your front knee.

3 When the watcher shouts "Everybody become a wise old owl!", point your elbows in the air, make circles with your middle finger and thumb, and place over your eyes. The first wise man to touch the watcher is the winner and becomes the watcher for the next round.

A yoga party

A yoga party can involve all members of the family and works particularly well with younger children. Use the yoga animal postures as your theme, and let them inspire your choice of decoration, party food and activity. Try some of the yoga games discussed earlier in this chapter, or try variations of more traditional games. Even better, make up some of your own.

Musical footsteps

Cut out footprint shapes to scatter on the dance floor. Start with enough pairs of feet for everyone, then take one foot away from each pair to have single feet only. Play lively music, and encourage everyone to dance about. When the music stops, everybody must stand on the footprints and make a yoga pose.

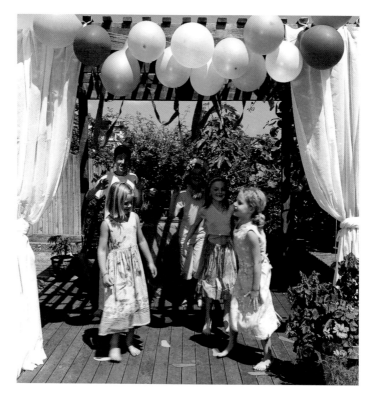

1 Place the pairs of footprints on the dance floor. Turn on the music and ask everyone to start dancing.

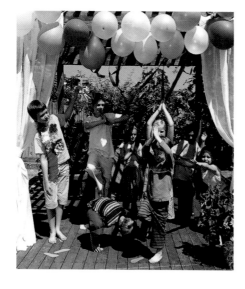

2 When the music stops everybody must jump on to a pair of footprints and adopt a yoga pose. Hold very still because if you wobble off your footprints you are out!

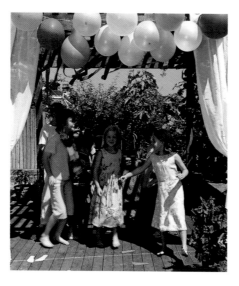

3 The children who are still in the game can start dancing when the music starts again. Meanwhile, take away one footprint from a few of the pairs.

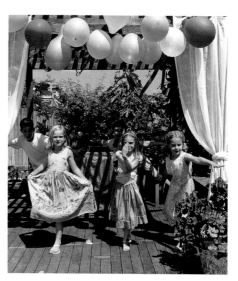

4 When the music stops this time, some children will have to balance on one leg. Continue taking away footprints until you have only one footprint and one winner.

Pass the parcel

Prepare a gift, wrapped in several layers of paper. All of you sit down in a circle and pass the parcel to one another using only your feet. When the music stops, you must tear off a layer with your toes. If you add a written forfeit between each layer of paper, you will have to perform a yoga pose when you remove the paper.

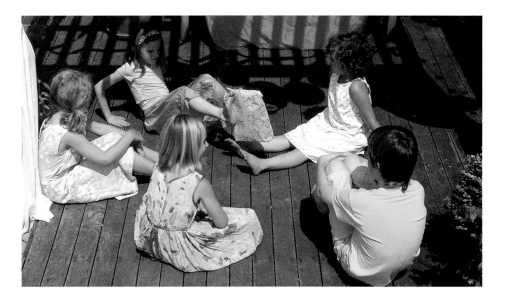

1 Everybody sits down in a circle on the floor. When the music begins, start to pass the parcel with your feet.

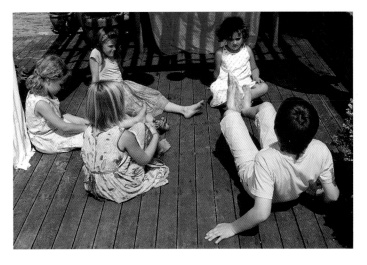

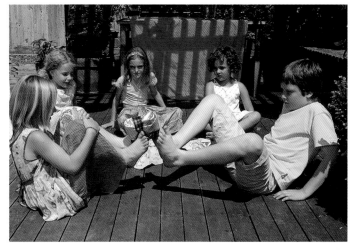

2 Keep on passing the parcel as long as the music is playing. Use your hands to support you and help you to keep your balance, but you can only pass the parcel with your feet.

3 When the music stops, whoever has the parcel must try to remove a layer of paper with their toes. Don't be tempted to use your hands or you will be out of the game!

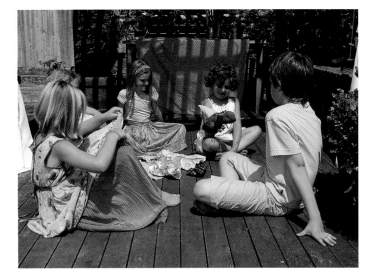

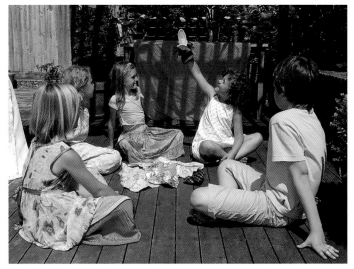

4 Whoever unwraps the final layer of paper is the winner, and is allowed to keep the special treat that they find inside.

5 You can add an extra dimension to the game by asking the winner to make a yoga pose based on the surprise they find inside the parcel.

▷

Bunny hopping

This relay race is great fun. Organize your guests into two teams (a minimum of three in each). Each child holds a balloon between their legs and must hop with a carrot baton in their mouth to the next child in the team. The baton is handed over and the next child sets off at full hop.

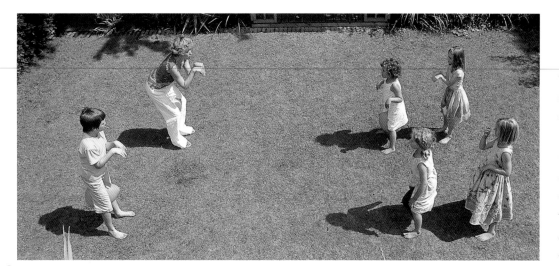

1 Take your positions with the two teams side by side. One bunny from each team stands facing their team at the other end of the garden. Make sure everyone has an inflated balloon in-between their knees. The first bunny in the line-up has the carrot baton in their mouth. On your marks, get set and GO! The first bunny sets off, hopping over to their opposite bunny team member.

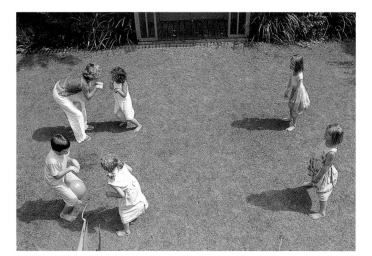

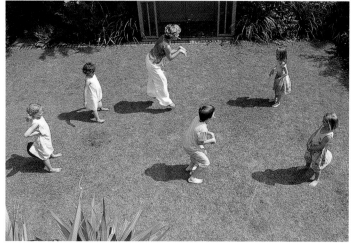

2 The first bunny of each team hops right across the garden towards the opposite bunny and makes the first exchange of the carrot baton. Take care not to let the balloons slip!

3 The first bunnies now stay where they are while the second bunnies set off hopping back across the garden to the rest of the team line-up, keeping the carrot batons in their mouths.

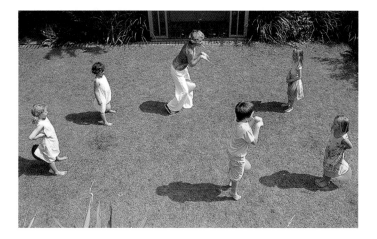

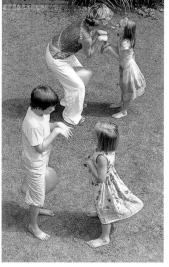

5 As the second bunnies reach the rest of their team they hand over the carrot baton for the final lap of the race.

4 Keep those legs springy and hold your hands up like rabbit paws as you hop across the garden.

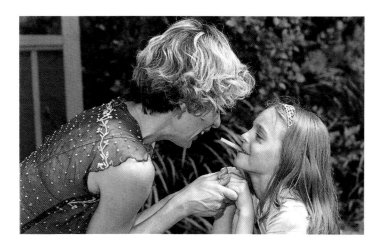

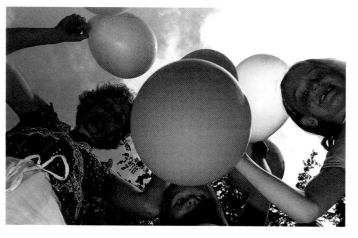

6 After exchanging batons, the third bunnies in the line-up now hop over to their opposite team members. The first team to hand over the carrot baton is the winner!

7 Wave your balloons in the air as the winning bunnies celebrate!

Party poppers

If your guests are still full of energy, get them to be party poppers, crouching down small to begin with, and preparing to spring up into the air with a high-energy burst. This should help to build up an appetite ready for the party food.

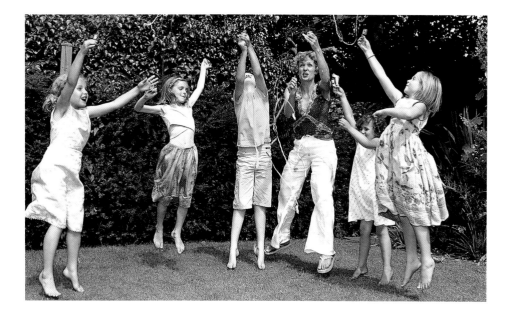

1 All crouch down small together and imagine you are a party popper filled with streamers and confetti and ready to explode. On a count of "1, 2, 3!" leap up into the air, stretching your arms as high as you can. If you like, you could let off party streamers as you jump up.

2 Come back down and repeat your leap all over again. Keep stretching your arms up high. Repeat as many times as you like until you can explode no more. Then all of you flop down together and rest.

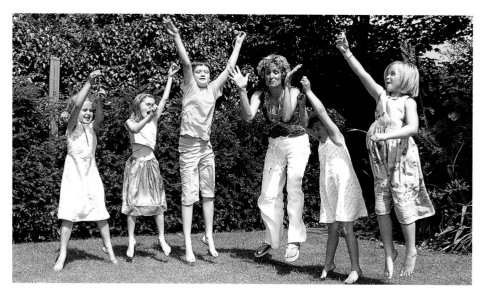

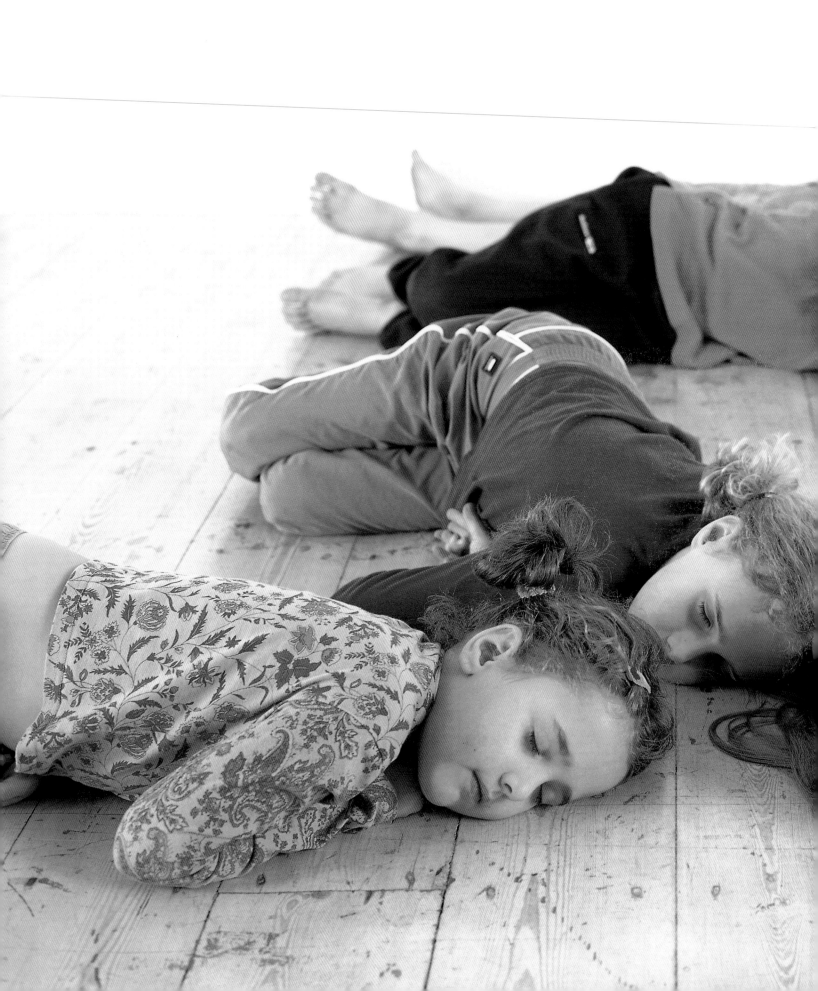

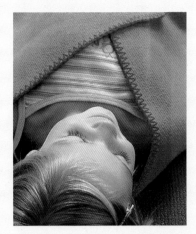

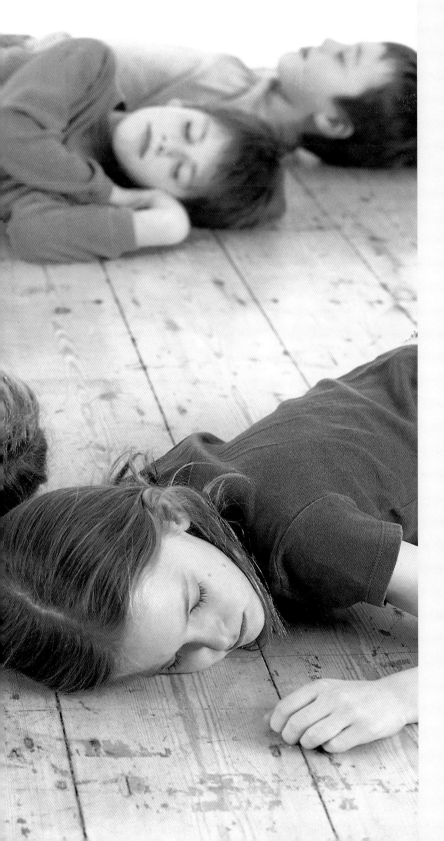

quiet
time

The appreciation of peace and quiet, the notion of *being* rather than *doing*, and the ability to jump off the merry-go-round of life and take time out are valuable life skills that we can all find beneficial. Enjoy these tranquil yoga postures when energy levels are low and you are in need of emotional nourishment, and learn how to appease everyday problems with simple, specially chosen postures.

Being quiet

Cultivating quiet time in our busy lives should be a weekly if not daily priority. Yoga teaches children to rediscover the joy of stillness and silence, and to see that being able to relax is just as important to health and well-being as exercise and activity.

These are a few simple exercises that can reconnect us with our breathing and encourage us to explore our senses. Being able to spend time in this contemplative state is a very important life skill, making us less reliant on external distractions, such as the television, and helping us to keep calm when life becomes frenetic.

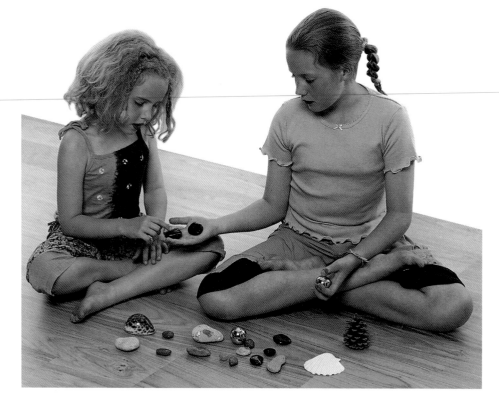

tummy breathing

Lie down in a quiet room in *shavasana* or Dead Man's pose. Place your hands or a soft toy on your tummy so that you can feel where your breath is and how it moves. Breathe deeply so that your tummy rises as you breathe in and falls as you breathe out. After about 5 minutes, roll to one side and slowly come up to a sitting position.

touchy feely

Our skin is a powerful sense organ. Simply touching objects with a pleasant surface can engender feelings of well-being. Stroking a pet, cuddling a soft teddy bear or exploring the surface of a pebble or sea shell encourages sensory awareness and a calm, contended state of mind.

△ Reacquainting yourself with special objects or treasures helps to rekindle happy memories and encourages contemplation.

Mala beads are used in traditional yoga practice to encourage inner contentment and mindfulness. The beads are held in the right hand and each bead is rolled between thumb and middle finger while a mantra (a special phrase or syllable) is repeated. You can use any string of beads instead of mala beads. Choose two words that are relevant to you. Sitting cross-legged with eyes closed, the beads can be rolled through the fingers while you repeat the word "Peace" on the in breath and "Calm" on the outward breath.

◁ Letting your mind rest on the ebb and flow of your natural breath is soothing and encourages physical stillness, which to a child can be the most challenging of all activities. Using a toy as a prop makes relaxation more fun.

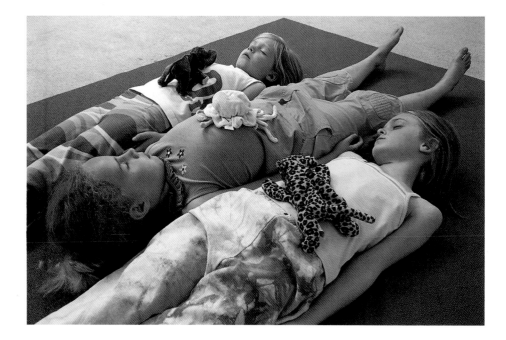

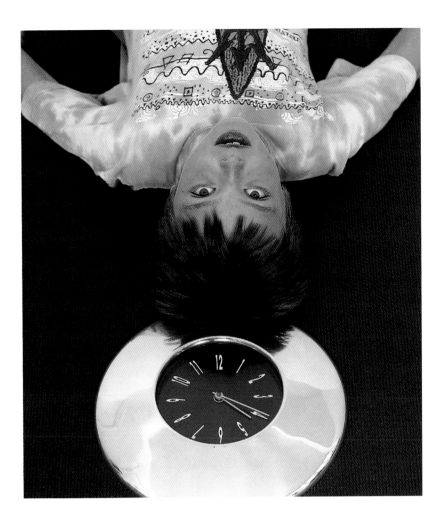

"Concentrate on silence.
When it comes, dwell on
what it sounds like. Then
strive to carry that quiet
wherever you go."

▽ Spend time encouraging connectedness.
Caring for special things at a young age can
develop a child's ability to care for others
later on in life, as well as showing her the
pleasures to be found in modest possessions.

simple sounds

Relaxing music is used instead of
medication in the treatment of some
stress-related illnesses and problems,
and often with tremendous success.
This testifies to the power of sound
and its effects on our well-being. On
the other hand, the wrong type of
sound can be damaging to our health.
The rumble of traffic in our cities,
constant background music piped
into shopping centres and the ringing
of phones both inside and outside the
home, can wear us down.

A breaking glass can shatter nerves
whereas bird song or the chiming
of bells can elicit positive feelings of
peace and joy. Everyday sounds, such
as the simple ticking of a clock, engage
our minds and, in turn, can improve
our ability to concentrate. As our
mind tunes in, our body gets a chance
to "chill out" for a while. Try writing
a list of the sounds you like, along
with another list of the sounds that
make you feel edgy or cross.

△ The gentle repetition of a pleasant and
familiar sound, such as a ticking wall clock,
can help to still a busy mind.

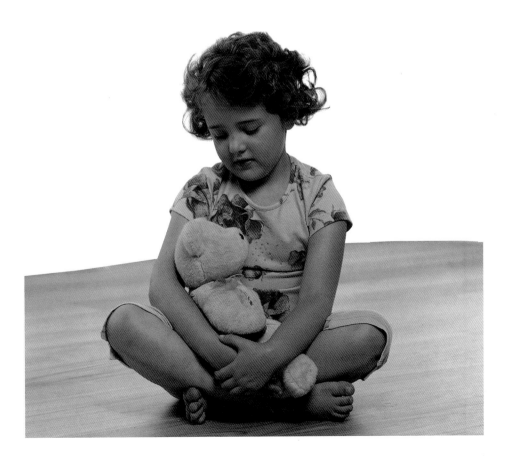

Peaceful postures

Poses that bring calm and tranquillity are restorative and rejuvenating to mind, body and soul. They are lovely to practise after a busy day or when you just feel like being quiet. You can practise them to wind yourself down after the energizing animal poses in the Animal Parade chapter, and done before bedtime they will ensure you get a sound and restful night's sleep.

Peaceful postures help to conserve your energy, rather than drain it out of your system. Even though you may feel you are doing very little as you practise them, you are actually doing something extremely powerful. You are recharging your internal batteries, rekindling your life force or *prana*, and this is what will keep you feeling full of energy, alive and well.

Many of the poses that bring a sense of peace to the body are done lying or sitting down with the eyes closed. The exceptions are the standing poses such as Tree pose, Mountain pose and Dancer. Concentration is needed to stand completely still. In doing so, we encourage our mind's internal chattering to fade away softly into the background.

▽ **Tree** Stand on one foot and lift the other up, placing the sole of your foot against your inner thigh. Bring your hands into prayer position or Namaste in front of you and steady yourself. Begin to feel your supporting foot spreading into the floor like imaginary roots growing down deep into the earth. Focus on a stationary point in front of you. Gently lift your arms above your head to form the branches of your tree. Feel strong and silent like a magnificent oak. Hold for a few deep breaths, then slowly release and change sides.

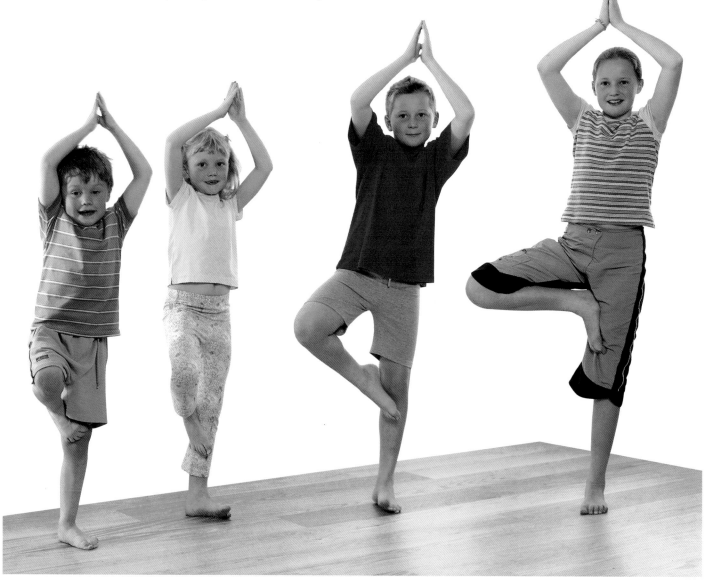

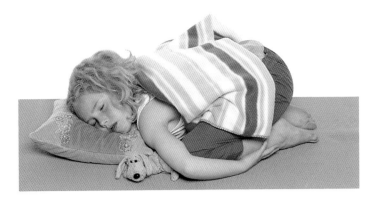

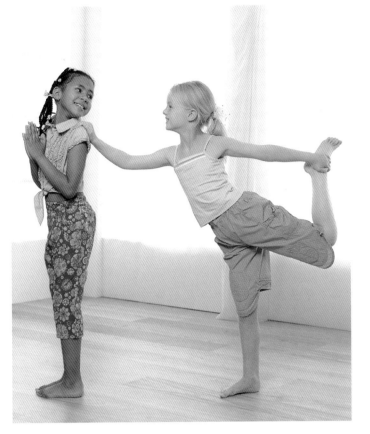

△ **Child's pose** Rest on your knees with your forehead on the floor or a cushion in front of you, arms by your sides. Picture a mouse curled up small and still, or a pebble on the beach, made smooth by the sea and warmed by the sun.

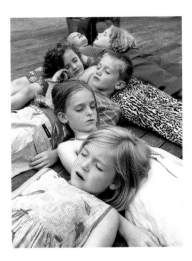

◁ **Sleeping snake** This is a lovely exercise for a group of friends. Lie down, one by one, with your head on the stomach of the person beneath you, forming a herringbone pattern. When assembled, close your eyes and feel your head gently lifting and dropping as the person you are resting on breathes in and out.

△ **Mountain and dancer** Feel as motionless as a mountain (left), with feet firm and an imaginary cord from the crown of your head helping you stand tall and proud. Face straight ahead to hold the position correctly. Dancer pose (right) requires a firm foot and an elegant grace.

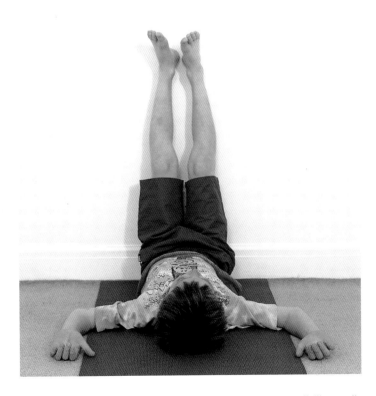

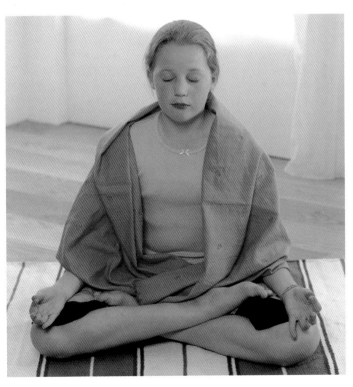

△ **Candle** Lying flat on your back with your legs up the wall, like a tall candle, gives legs a rest from the effects of gravity. Stretch your arms above your head, close your eyes and breathe deeply. Imagine a cool waterfall refreshing your legs and whole body.

△ **Little Buddha** Sitting with the legs crossed ensures your spine is anchored and that you are able to sit tall and straight. With your hands in your lap or resting on the knees you can feel strength and wisdom growing inside you. This is the classic pose of meditation.

Dream time

Dream time is simply deep relaxation for children. This is a time when you lie completely still, allowing your body to relax and switch off for a while. With regular practice and encouragement, you will come to look forward to this part of your yoga session, particularly if you aim to make it special.

preparation

To make the dream time session more fun, put some thought into getting ready. Think about the music you would like to listen to and allow yourself one special toy that can lie down with you while you dream.

Select a favourite cushion or blanket and make yourself feel as warm and comfortable as possible. The best time for dream time is towards the end of the day, when your energy levels are naturally low, and fading light and the prospect of bedtime makes you want to feel cosy and snug. You can either practise dream time after your active yoga poses or on its own as an extra special dream session, especially if you are feeling tired.

the rewards of stillness

Children can be offered a simple reward for stillness if they are unable to concentrate on being quiet –

for example, a pretty pebble, shell, wild flower, feather or crystal. Younger children can be told that a visiting fairy or elf will place something nice in their hands but only when they are completely still and quiet. This small incentive can work wonders.

dead man pose

The classic yoga relaxation pose is *shavasana*, also known as Corpse pose or Dead Man pose. The body lies still, with the feet hip-width apart, the arms away from the body and the eyes closed. Resting in *shavasana* allows the body to rest and recharge depleted energy stores.

sweet dreams

- Choose a quiet room, turn off the lights and light a few candles (but do not leave these burning unattended). Make your children comfortable with cushions, pillows, blankets and any toys or props.
- Put on some soothing music – natural sounds such as bird song, waves or rainfall, soft drums or pipes usually work best.
- As they lie on their backs, ask children to feel really heavy. As gravity gently draws them down into the ground, let them feel their body melting like ice cream.
- Do the "spaghetti" test. Gently go round to each child and lift one leg or arm at a time and tell them to make it feel really heavy. This will show that they are starting to relax. Rock the limb gently from side to side, then place it carefully back on the floor.

- Ask the child to think about their breathing and whereabouts in their bodies their breath is. Ask them to feel their tummies moving up and down as they breathe in and out. They could try to imagine a tiny boat at sea, bobbing up and down gently on the ocean waves.
- Tell them to relax their feet, repeating, "Relax my feet, my feet are heavy and r-e-l-a-x-e-d", and continue for each part of the body right up to their head.
- Tell them how difficult it is to be still and how clever they are to resist moving. Remind them that their ability to relax is a special gift.
- Visually guide them on a special journey. Let their yoga mat become a flying carpet gliding over a tropical rainforest or a soft cloud passing through a rainbow. Or take them to a golden beach where they can feel the warm yellow sand underneath their

feet, and hear the playful call of dolphins inviting them to come and swim. Choose a theme, using your imagination, and keep the language simple. Allow time for them to explore their "dream".
- When your child looks relaxed and still, introduce a simple affirmation or resolve, such as "I feel free and happy!". Ask them to repeat it to themselves three times. Pause for a moment and then gently guide them back to reality. Tell them they are waking up in bed and ask them to gently stretch and yawn.
- When they are ready, ask them to talk about their dream and share it with you.

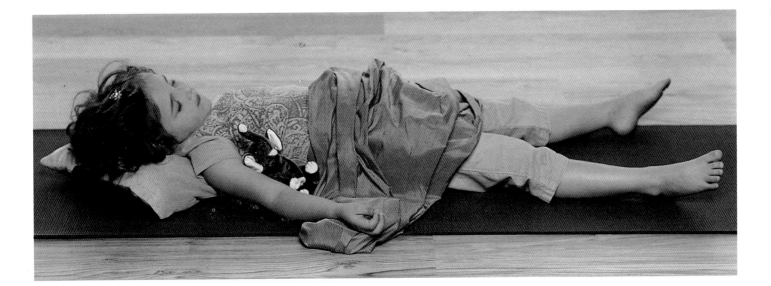

△ **Shavasana** Praise your child for lying motionless and resisting the urge to move. Tell her that in doing so her mind is being taken on a wonderful holiday.

special time

Many important physiological changes take place in *shavasana*. Respiration levels are lowered, strain on the heart is reduced and the vital life energy, or *prana*, that has been created in posture work can be assimilated into the body. As the breath quietens and softens, the mind becomes clear and detached. It is then receptive to any positive images or sounds you may hear.

making a resolve

Relaxation encourages the mind to be open and receptive. It is therefore a wonderful time to be introduced to positive ideas and images in the form of an affirmation or *sankalpa*. These little seeds of hope will embed themselves in your consciousness over time, and can help you to feel good about yourself. Affirmations should only ever be simple, even for older

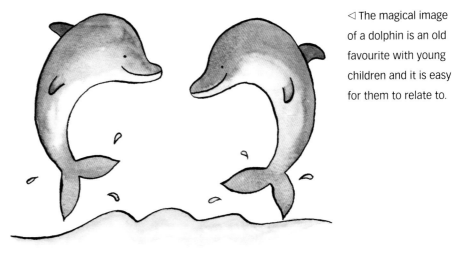

◁ The magical image of a dolphin is an old favourite with young children and it is easy for them to relate to.

children, and negative words and images should be avoided as these can be counter productive. Choose one affirmation for the session, and repeat it in your head three times.

▽ If you are talking a child through their dream, keep the images and words that you use light, sunny and positive.

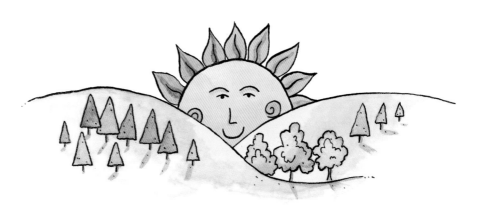

Sounding it out

Sound is an invisible yet powerful form of energy created by the vibration of molecules. Adding sound to your yoga practice encourages self-expression and develops good communications skills. Sighing, humming or chanting also helps to put us in touch with the quiet place inside us, where new sensations and emotions can be experienced.

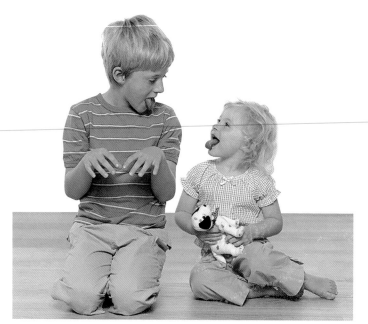

◁ Imitating animals and the sounds they make is a fun and creative part of your yoga practice.

animal antics

Everyone will enjoy panting like a dog, sniffing like a rabbit, hissing like a snake or roaring like a lion as they practise the animal poses in the Animal Parade chapter. Get really involved and make sounds and movements to elaborate on the pose.

humming bee breath

This breath helps to open up the throat chakra, which is the centre of communication. It can help to dissolve the fear of speaking up at school to teachers, and will help when speaking to new friends. To do the Humming Bee Breath, sit in Little Buddha pose with your eyes closed. Breathe in and as you breathe out through your mouth, gently hum at the same time. Feel the sound gently vibrating in your throat.

Try putting your fingers in your ears as you hum to really help you concentrate and feel the sound resonating deep within you.

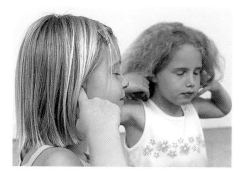

△ ▽ Removing the distractions of external noises by putting fingers in your ears can help to put you in touch with your inner world.

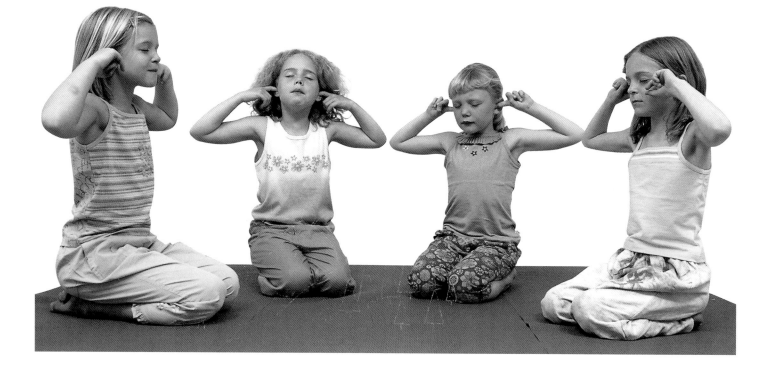

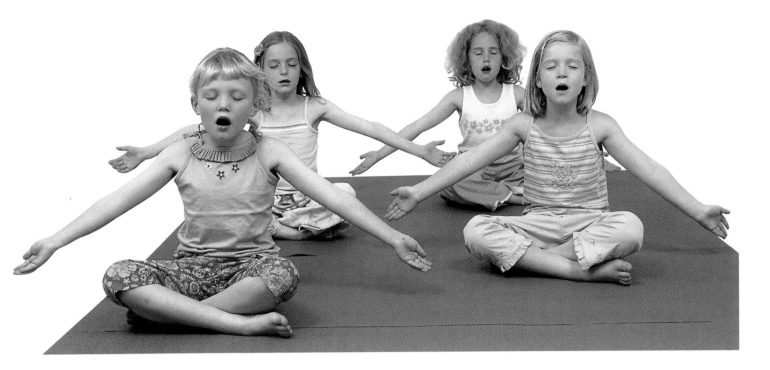

sighing breath

This breath helps you to let go of stresses and strains at the end of a busy day. First breathe in deeply, then sigh the breath out of your mouth with a lovely strong "Aaaahh!" sound. Repeat a few times and now visualize anything that has made you cross or sad floating out with your breath and up and away into space.

chanting

Yogic chanting is a form of singing or humming and produces special vibrations that soothe body, mind and soul. A mantra is a special word that can be hummed as you chant.

Om is the classic yoga mantra – meaning absolute peace. The wise yogis believed that we should "live in Om". In other words, we should live our lives in total peace and harmony.

Begin by repeating Om in your head, breaking it down into three sections. Start with an "Ah" sound, then an "Oh" sound then "Mmmm". Then breathe in and, as you breathe

▷ Sighing out through the mouth brings a sense of relief and helps you let go of unwanted feelings.

out, hum the Om out nice and loudly, visualizing each syllable as a little bubble of energy growing inside you and floating up into the sky. Try lifting your arms up slowly as you hum it to help your energy bubbles float upwards. Pause after each "Om" and see if you can hear or feel the echo of Om in your mind, and maybe in your body, too, as the sound waves keep on vibrating through you.

△ Chanting "Om" with our friends bonds us together. It makes us feel good about ourselves and makes friendships stronger.

You can also make up your own mantras, choosing a word relevant to how you are feeling. Evocative words such as "Peace", "Calm" or "Love" work very well. Let their soothing tones suffuse into every molecule of your body.

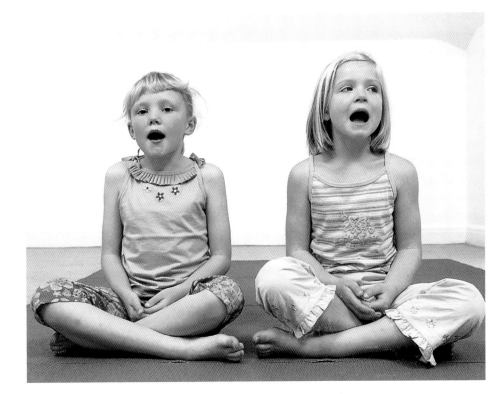

The wise yogi

Yoga is often referred to as "skill in action". This defines not just the physical skills that yoga provides us with, but also the mental skills that teach us control of our mind and our emotions.

Establishing these skills helps us to understand our true nature, and this gives us more control over our lives. Getting to know and accept our strengths and weaknesses gives us a sort of inner power and equips us with a code for living. This helps us to manage the up and downs of daily life more easily and with confidence.

Being able to help yourself and the rest of your family overcome everyday ailments and upsets is a wonderful example of how yoga gives us better control over our lives. In addition to the physical advantages of yoga practice, you can learn how to use the postures therapeutically and holistically to make yourself feel better.

▽ **Wheel** Prepare your back by doing Blue Whale pose a few times. Then lie in the same starting position tuck your flat palms under your shoulders. Breathe deeply and on a breath out, push strongly into your hands and lift your bottom and head off the floor. Hold for a few breaths, then release and hug your knees.

headaches

Forward bends can help to relieve everyday headaches. The act of leaning forwards also helps to still the mind and lessen the load on the heart. In a darkened room, try Child's pose with your head on a cushion, or Sandwich pose supporting your head and arms with a chair. Close your eyes and breathe calmly for 5–10 minutes.

low energy

Back bends are energizing as they open the heart and lungs, allowing us to breathe deeply. They also strengthen the nervous system and stimulate the digestive organs, improving the elimination of waste products. Try Cobra, Fish or Locust poses, or simply lie over a bean bag, arching your back. Take long breaths. For a really strong back bend, try doing Wheel pose.

stiffness and tension

Aches in the lower back can be caused by many things from slouching to carrying heavy loads, or strenuous

"Yoga helps to cure what need not be endured and to endure what cannot be cured"

physical activity. You can find relief by lying on your back and hugging your knees in tightly to you chest. Rocking forwards and backwards helps massage the back muscles, "ironing" away strain and tension. Child's pose, Beetle and Blue Whale are also very effective. To maintain spinal mobility and strength, practise Sunshine Stretch and Cat, Dog, Snake and Mouse.

tummy ache

Lie on your front allowing the floor to gently cushion your tummy. Breathe deep breaths to let your tummy relax.

sore throat

Roaring Lion is good for keeping sore throats at bay. It is also guaranteed to bring a smile to the face of anyone in a bad mood. Practised in a group, it encourages team work.

nerves

Woodchopper pose or Roaring Lion help to release pent up energy and nervousness, particularly before an important event.

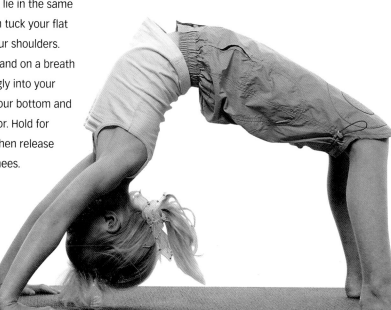

asthma

With commitment, yoga can help you to manage and even control the symptoms of bronchial asthma. Regular practice strengthens the respiratory system, drains mucus from the lungs, promotes breath awareness and control, and relaxes tense chest muscles. Gentle movements, which encourage rhythmic breathing, are good for asthma sufferers; aggressive movements may over-stimulate the lungs. Try Sunshine Stretch to get the whole body moving, and gentle back bends to relax the chest.

A breathing exercise such as Sniffing Breath can be useful. Sit quietly with crossed legs. Bring your mind to your breath and breathe naturally for a few moments. Then begin to sniff as you breathe in, taking two or three short sniffing breaths until the lungs are full, then a long breath out. Repeat until your chest feels open and relaxed. This also helps if you have been upset or crying.

hyperactivity

Strong poses and animal postures with accompanying noises will use up excess energy and disperse physical tension. Follow with some of the breathing techniques, such as Sighing Breath or Humming Bee Breath to soothe and relax.

▽ **Supported back bend** Arching your body backwards over an exercise ball or bean bag makes you feel wide awake. Not having to support your own weight means you can relax and hold the pose for longer.

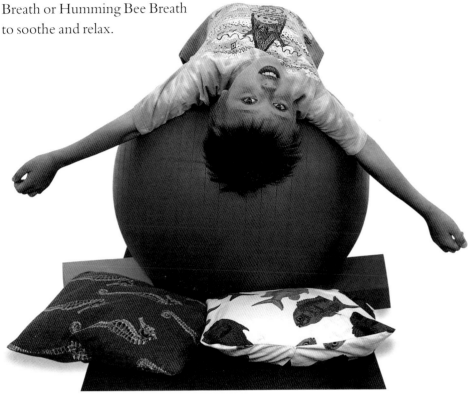

Shoulder stand

This calming pose revives you after a busy day and reverses the effects of gravity on the legs and heart. Close your eyes and visualize a refreshing mountain waterfall pouring energy back into your legs. For a milder version, lie sideways against a wall, and extend your legs so that they rest against the wall. Take your arms to the floor behind your head and relax completely for 5 minutes.

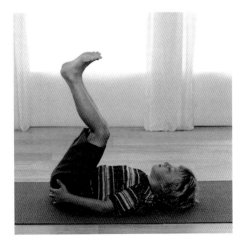

1 Lie on your back on the floor and lift your legs upwards, with your knees bent. Keep your chin tucked in towards your chest to protect your neck.

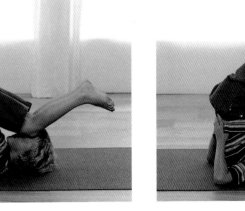

2 With your hands on your lower back, drop the knees down towards your face. This will allow your back to peel off the floor. You can support your back with your hands.

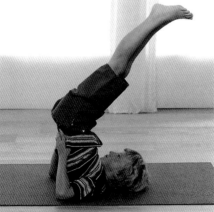

3 Lift your legs upwards as you push your lower back towards your face with your hands. Close your eyes and breathe. Roll your back down on to the floor. Hug your knees.

▷

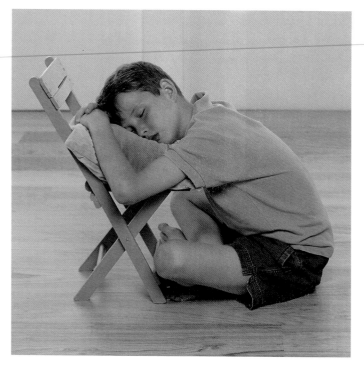

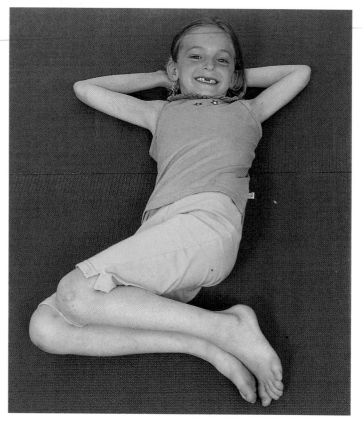

△ **Forward bend with chair** This lovely relaxing pose requires no effort and helps to quieten a busy mind or an aching head.

▽ **Canny cat** Cat pose is a very versatile pose and it is fun and easy to do. Get down on your hands and knees and roar like a big cat or tuck your toes under, lift up your bottom and become a dog. Become a cat again, then sit on your heels and be quiet again in Child's pose.

△ **Easy twist** To ease a strained or aching back, lie on your back, knees bent and feet flat on the floor. Interlace your fingers under your head and, as you breathe out, let your knees drop to one side. Hold for five deep breaths and change sides. Feel your back waking up.

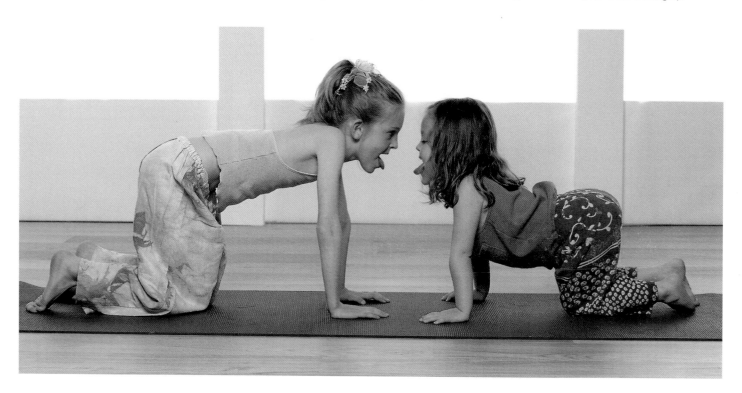

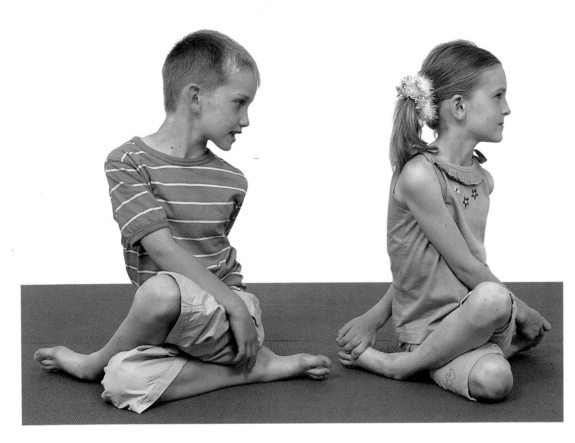

◁ **Seated twist** Twisting poses help to unravel knots or tight bits in your back and, according to yoga therapists, any knots or problems in your head too. Sit cross-legged with your left leg on the top. Slide this leg over so that your knees are almost on top of one another and your left heel is by your right thigh. Breathe in and lift your chest. Then breathe out and turn your body to the left. Let your spine spiral round, from the bottom upwards. Place your right arm on your left thigh and try to catch your left toes with your left hand. Change sides after a few deep breaths.

▷ **Sweet dreams**
The yogis believed that stilling the eyes and focusing our gaze or *drushti* would help to focus the mind. Learn to relax with a prop. A soothing, lavender eye bag or silk scarf will help you to keep inquisitive, seaching eyes closed.

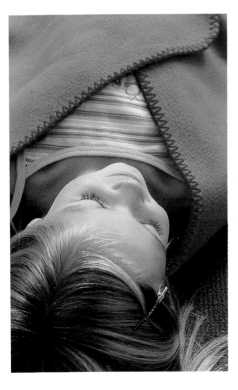

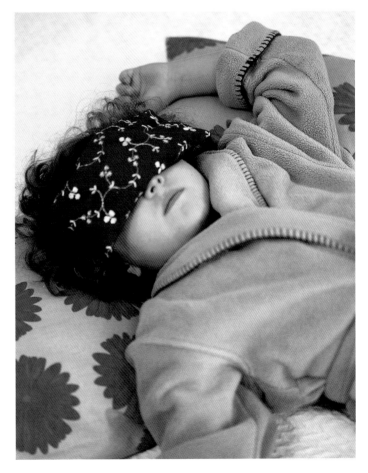

△ **Shavasana** "I closed my eyes so I could see". Just a few quiet moments lying down wrapped in a cosy blanket can help you to feel calm and good about yourself again.

Index

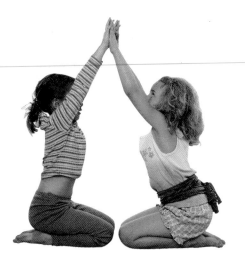

acknowledgements

The Author and Publishers would like to thank the children who modelled for this book:
Laurie Ainscough, Kari-Ann Barbe Parker, Esme Chapman, Leah Chapman, Luke Chapman, Pascal Clark, Max Crowther, Megan Crowther, Chiron D'Antal, Georgia Gibbs, Brittany Gibbs, Lauren Hobbs, Siena Hobbs, Josh Kean, Sam Kean, Alex Knight, Ella Knight, Rosie Knight, Hannah Lie, Nicholas Lie, Oliver Man, Abigail Marrow, Alex Marrow, Ben Marrow, Elspie Marrow, Jo Mayda, Beau McCarthy, Jack Reid, Nicola Reid, Do-Do Schleppers, Folkert Schleppers, Tina Schleppers, Jamie Skinner Powell, Alex Woodman, Bryony Wood, James Woodman and Leo Zunz.

Thanks also to the following companies for lending us beautiful clothes for photography:
Oilily,
9 Sloane Street,
London SW1X GLE
Tel. 020 7823 2505

Adore Mail Order,
Tel. 0906 302 0321 for a catalogue or log on to *www.adorelondon.co.uk*.